Everyday Wholesome Eating

In the Raw

By Kim Wilson

cost-effective and time-efficient
raw food recipes for everyday people

Whether you're just interested in adding more raw foods
to your diet to boost your nutritional intake
or seriously considering becoming a "raw foodist",
within these pages you'll find an immense variety
of recipes that are tasty and easy to prepare.

Everyday Wholesome Eating In the Raw

Fourth Edition
© Copyright 2012 by Kim Wilson
Lebanon, NH
All rights reserved

See more of the *Everyday Wholesome Eating* series at:
www.simplynaturalhealth.com

Cover Design by Linnea Lewis

ISBN 978-0-9831312-4-3

First Printing 2002
Second Printing 2007
Third Printing 2009
Printed in the United States of America

Table of Contents

Introductory Information

The Benefits of Raw Foods

Raw foods come to us with the living **enzymes** necessary to facilitate the digestion and assimilation of the nutrients in the foods. Cooking kills all enzymes, as well as most vitamins, and alters the minerals and proteins in such a way that they are less usable to the body. Because the cooked food is not accompanied by the enzymes necessary for digestion, it places more of a strain on our digestive system and many of the nutrients that are left after cooking are lost in this process (besides those lost through any refining or processing).

Raw foods are also the most **nutritionally dense** because all of the original vitamins, minerals, proteins, fats and fiber are in their unaltered forms and completely available to our bodies. A raw food offers up to three times the nutrition of the same cooked. Since true nutrition is concerned with feeding our cells, it is important to provide them with the living nutrients of raw foods. Life can be sustained on cooked foods, but cells are not replenished and replaced in an optimal way. On raw foods you will find that you eat less, yet your body will operate more efficiently with what you provide. Also because raw foods are **easily digested**, less energy will be expended on the process of digestion and be available to you for other activities. Most people who add more raw foods to their diet are surprised by the increase in energy they experience.

Live foods feed a living body.

Reasons for RAW

1. When we eat raw foods we are consuming them as close to the way they were originally created as possible.
2. **All** animals subsist on an all raw diet (*except* for humans and their pets)
3. Raw foods are in their purest state (organic) Unaltered by heat, chemicals, stabilizers, preservatives, colorings, additives, etc.
4. Packed with nutrients in most body-available forms:

Amino acids	Phytochemicals
Essential fatty acids	Antioxidants
Complex carbohydrates	Chlorophyll
Vitamins	Fiber
Minerals	Purified water
Enzymes	Oxygen

5. Raw diet provides more vitamins, minerals, antioxidants, phytonutrients (etc.), than any other diet!
6. In contrast, cooking:
   a. Destroys oxygen, enzymes and chlorophyll
   b. Destroys a great portion of vitamins
   c. Alters minerals (rendered inorganic)
   d. Alters/harms fats and fiber
   e. Requires more energy for digestion
      cooked foods - 35-65% of energy
      raw foods- 8-12% of energy
   f. Requires more time for digestion (2-3x)
   g. Encourages overeating- because nutritional content is lacking, our cells are still looking for nutrition.

Other Nice Side-Benefits
Of Consuming Raw Foods

Convenience   Raw food meals can be very simple to prepare (you can't get much easier than an all-fruit lunch!), and the clean-up is even easier.   No soaking or scrubbing pans with cooked-on food or cleaning a stovetop.

Less hygienic issues   Body odor, phlegm, bad breath and tartar build-up on your teeth will not be the problems they are on a cooked-food diet.

Less health issues   Raw foods naturally support our optimal health because they are consumed as close to the way they were originally created as possible.   They do not cause or support illness or degenerative disease.   Eating raw also allows us more mental clarity.

Natural weight maintenance   Whether you are overweight and need to shed a few pounds or underweight and need to gain a few, raw foods allow your body to normalize to its correct weight and maintain it year in and out. *That's a nice side-benefit!*

Keeps appetite in check   Raw foods satisfy with less. Cooked foods, in contrast, stimulate our appetite and encourage us to overeat on nutrient-robbed foods.

Great source of clean, pure water   We don't have to obsess over how much water we're taking in when we're consuming raw foods so rich in naturally distilled water.

Undiscovered benefits of raw foods   Considering the fact that the nutritional components we do know about (vitamins, minerals, protein, fats, enzymes, . . .) are injured, altered or destroyed by heating, we should ask ourselves what other benefits might we be unknowingly missing out on by cooking our foods.

Food combining is simplified   When eating cooked foods, principles of food combining are important to follow to limit digestive problems.   (Basic principles: Proteins and starches can be eaten with non-starchy vegetables, but not with each other. Fruits should always be eaten on their own). Food combining becomes less of an issue when consuming all raw foods. This means you can be more flexible with adding fruits to salads, for instance.

Food allergies/sensitivities become less of a problem These are most often the body's response to refined, processed and cooked foods.   It's much easier to avoid problematic foods when concentrating on raw foods.   For instance, it's super easy to eat gluten-free this way!

Foods that are normally problematic don't tend to be in their raw form   For example, foods like honey and vinegar that are often a problem for people with candida are rarely so when consumed in their whole, natural, raw form.

The Important Role of Enzymes

-enzymes are naturally abundant in raw foods-

Enzymes are the **"passports"** that effectively get nutrients to where they are needed in the body. It is futile to calculate a food's nutritional value based on the vitamin, mineral, protein, fat and carbohydrate content if the enzymes have been rendered powerless by the cooking process. If the nutritional components themselves have been altered or destroyed by the heating, then even what remains won't be able to get effectively where it needs to go without their guides- the enzymes.

Enzymes convert

- fats and oils into simple fatty acids
- complex carbohydrates into simple sugars
- proteins into amino acids

Heating foods above 105-118 degrees destroys the enzymes.

In order to digest cooked foods a great deal of energy plus the sacrifice of some of the body's nutritional reserves are required by the body to compensate for the lack of enzymes.

Raw Foods/Living Foods

Raw foods are simply unheated, uncooked foods. Many raw foods aren't truly living, however since they aren't actively involved in the growth process.

Living foods are alive because they are growing. They contain a "life force"- energy able to support life. Living foods are those that have been newly harvested, or those to which new growth has been activated through soaking or sprouting. Examples of live foods are freshly harvested fruits and vegetables, freshly-grown sprouts, and soaked or sprouted nuts, seeds, grains or legumes.

Cooked vs. Raw Fats/Oils

Heating fats changes their chemical composition. This complicates our body's work in assimilating this substance. Fats in their raw, natural form, however, are efficiently used by the body and are highly beneficial.

Whereas we normally think of fats as "fattening", raw fats can actually be beneficial for healthy weight maintenance. Research shows that coconut oil contains a unique form of fatty acid that stimulates metabolism, gives you more energy, and promotes weight loss, among other things.

Raw oils (like coconut oil) are also great applied directly to the skin.

Truly Raw?

Many seemingly raw ingredients aren't so because of the processing or drying process they have gone through. Be sure to find a reliable source for raw ingredients. The best way to test for 'rawness' of beans, legumes, grains, and seeds is to attempt to sprout them.

Some Foods That Aren't Necessarily Raw

Tahini "Shelf-stable" means it was heated in processing.

Coconut Shredded coconut has usually been pasteurized and/or dried at questionable temperatures.

Honey Honey is usually pasteurized and filtered. The label needs to read "raw" or "unheated" for it to be truly raw.

Oats Rolled oats are steamed in the processing and most oat groats are heated to stabilize them. You can attempt to soak and sprout some oat groats to test whether they are raw or not. I don't choose to use oat groats in my raw recipes because I don't find the finished product as appetizing. If you choose to use oat groats you can substitute them for buckwheat groats in some of the recipes.

Figs, dates, prunes Sometimes steamed.

Spice blends Often toasted or roasted.

Olives Unless they have been salt or oil-cured, they have been cooked.

Tips for Transitioning to a Diet That Includes More and More Raw Foods

Concentrate on adding more raw foods to your diet (rather than focusing on eliminating cooked foods) In time, raw foods automatically replace cooked foods.

1. Enjoy fruit for a snack

2. Begin cooked meals with a large salad

3. Eat one raw meal per day
   - Fresh fruit or vegetable juices for breakfast
   - An all-fruit breakfast
   - An all-fruit lunch

4. Increase, in time, to 2 raw meals per day
   Breakfast- Fresh fruit or vegetable juices,
      or an all-fruit meal
   Lunch or dinner- all-fruit meal, salads or raw entrees
   Even try a "dessert dinner"! Start off with a fruit smoothie or soft-serve ice cream, then top it off with a pie or fruit-and-nut truffles. What a treat!

5. On occasion, try an all-raw or all-fruit day (especially when you are ill or cleansing)

Note: *Most people find they do best on a predominantly raw (not exclusively raw) diet. An all-raw diet can be difficult to maintain for various reasons. You'll find you have more flexibility and that social connections are easier to maintain with a diet that includes both raw and cooked foods. Some foods (like beans and grains) are also much more palatable in cooked form. Some people with compromised digestion also will find they need to go slowly when adding more raw foods to their diet, allowing time for their system to adjust and heal.*

Changes

As your health improves with more raw foods,
you'll probably notice a few new changes

Your tastes change. You develop a greater desire for foods that are good for you.

You require smaller amounts of food. The foods you consume are more nutrient-dense and your digestion and assimilation have improved.

You desire simple foods. You come to savor salads and enjoy simple foods all on their own or in simple combinations, like fruit and nuts.

Why Use a Dehydrator?

Dehydrated foods (crackers, cookies, snacks) offer some of the familiar flavors, crunch and warmth of cooked foods. Dehydrating also allows for long-term storage of foods.

A dehydrator can also be used to warm a recipe/dish.
Raw foods don't need to be served cold
Simply allow a dish to sit out for a few hours to warm up to room temperature   **-or-**
Place on bottom shelf of dehydrator (don't stress the trays with a heavy dish) at 100 degrees for 2-6 hours.

Though a dehydrator can be a useful tool in preparing raw foods, I would place it low on the wish-list of kitchen tools.

Helpful Kitchen Tools for Raw Food Prep

Simple Basics

Wooden cutting board   *Designate one side for onions and garlic and the other for fruit and vegetables. Just rinse and allow to dry thoroughly between uses – no need for soap.*

Small knife   *For peeling and cutting up smaller items*

Large knife (chef's knife)   *For chopping larger items*

Vegetable peeler

Garlic press

Glass storage bowls with covers

½ pint, pint and quart size canning jars   *For storing juice, nuts, seeds, grains, etc. and for soaking/sprouting ingredients*

Very helpful appliances/tools

Food processor
For grating, slicing, grinding, chopping and pureeing.

Heavy-duty blender
For processing dressings and sauces, and for blending nuts, seeds and other firm raw ingredients

Dehydrator
For preserving foods and for making crisp or chewy recipes- crackers, cookies, cereals, fruit leathers, etc.

Juicer   *For making fresh vegetable and fruit juices, ice cream, etc.*

Salad spinner

Citrus juicer

Coffee grinder
For grinding flax seed primarily, but can be used for grinding other seeds and some herbs/spices

Mandoline slicer
For thinly slicing vegetables for chips, lasagna, etc.

Spiral slicer
For cutting veggies into pasta-like threads

Tips for Use of Appliances

Heavy-duty blender Include at least 3-4 cups of ingredients for thorough processing. Always keep plunger in (if blender comes with one) to circulate ingredients and prevent air bubbles from forming.

Mandoline slicer To prevent screw from loosening (and blade from slipping), cover screw with plastic wrap before putting into place.

Dehydrator Use parchment paper on dehydrating sheets for mixtures that are thin or small enough that they would fall through the mesh. Regularly set your dehydrator at 100 degrees, then you won't have to ask yourself, "Now, at what temperature is this supposed to be?" When dehydrating you are interested in retaining the living enzymes and nutrition, and 100 degrees is a safe temperature for doing so. (Be sure to check the accuracy of your dehydrator temperature with a thermometer).

Juicer Be sure to purchase a quality masticating juicer (where the fruits and vegetables are ground and pressed), not a centrifugal juicer (where the produce is cut and thrown in a spinning basket). The quality of the juice and preservation of the enzymes and nutrition in a masticating juicer is far superior. You will also be able to store the juice from a masticating juicer (that from a centrifugal juicer needs to be consumed immediately).

Goals for Raw Recipes

Simple- limited ingredients and steps.

Easy preparation- minimal appliances/tools, time, ingredients, and complexity.

Easy clean-up- using a limited number of dishes and kitchen equipment.

Focused on good foods- centering our meals on fruits and vegetables that we want to include in our diet. Limiting amount of grains, legumes, nuts and seeds- these richer foods should comprise a smaller portion of our diet.

Cost-effective- limiting the amounts of high cost ingredients (reserving for special occasion dishes).

Time-efficient- raw food prep shouldn't be more time-consuming than cooked food prep.

Good variety of quick-prep dishes- a balance of quick recipes and those (particularly dehydrated recipes) that require beginning a day or more ahead.

Focused on using real, familiar, whole foods - to create simple dishes that appeal to or are familiar enough to American/popular tastes, though not necessarily attempting to reproduce familiar cooked foods.

Raw Prep Methods

Size/Texture
- whole
- cut
- sliced
- diced
- chopped
- grated

Moisture
- dry
- soaked
- sprouted
- dehydrated

Processor
- chop
- grind
- puree

Temperature
- room temp.
- warm (dehydr.)
- cold (refrig.)
- frozen (freezer)

Blender
- puree
- smooth

These treatments are important to consider because they can drastically change the flavor and texture of an ingredient. For instance, soaked almonds seem similar to coconut in texture and flavor, in contrast to unsoaked raw almonds which are oilier and have a stronger flavor. Frozen bananas have a very mild flavor, yet bananas added to a dehydrated recipe can easily become overpowering.

Soaked nuts/seeds- will lend a creamy texture and flavor to a recipe.

Unsoaked nuts/seeds- process into a granular and more oily texture.

Lifespan of Prepared Raw Foods

Foods prepared with lemon juice and apple cider vinegar have a significantly longer lifespan. Dressings, dips, etc. can keep at least 1 week and up to 2 weeks in the refrigerator.

Tahini prepared from sesame seeds, sea salt and olive oil will keep for up to one month in the refrigerator.

It's always best to store foods you are not using in the refrigerator, but foods that you will soon be serving don't need to be kept cold in the refrigerator. If the food would be more pleasing at room temperature or warmer, take it out several hours prior to serving and let it sit on a counter or place in dehydrator. Our 'hang- ups' with letting food sit out is founded in our experience with animal-based foods (meats, dairy, mayonnaise, etc.) that invite the growth of microorganisms at room temperature and above.

Dehydrated Foods

I prefer to keep seeds, nuts and grains whole before dehydrating. Cutting them exposes the oils and opens them to decomposition. That's why, for instance, I use whole flax seeds in making flax crackers.
I only use ground flax in recipes that are going to be consumed immediately (not stored or dehydrated).
I also prefer to refrigerate all my dehydrated foods for further protection.

Food Qualities

Sweet
Honey
Dates, Raisins
Dried Apricots, Figs
Apples
Bananas
Dried fruit
Carob powder
Cinnamon

Sour
Lemon juice
Apple cider vinegar
Cranberries

Salty
Unrefined sea salt
Celery
Sea vegetables

Oily
Olive oil
Coconut oil
Nuts/Seeds
Avocado

Crunchy
Cut/sliced vegetables
Dehydrated chips/crackers

Creamy
Sunflower seeds
Pumpkin seeds
Tahini
Macadamias
Pine nuts
Soaked almonds
Avocado
Coconut oil

Thickening
Psyllium powder
Flax and chia seeds
Nuts/seeds

Meaty Texture
Chopped nuts
Ground seeds

Dairy-like
Sour cream/yogurt-
    Sunflower seeds/lemon
Cream cheese-
    Nuts/lemon/honey
Sharpness-
    Tahini/lemon/salt

Tomato paste-like
Sun-dried tomatoes

Raw Materials
For Raw Food Preparation

Fruits

Lemons
Oranges
Grapefruit

Kiwi
Pineapple
Mango
Papaya

Grapes
Strawberries
Blueberries
Raspberries
Cranberries

Apples
Pears
Peaches
Plums
Bananas
Melons

Dried Fruits

Raisins
Prunes
Apricots
Figs
Dates
Apples
Papaya
Tomatoes

Be sure all dried fruits are dried at low temperatures and are unsweetened and unsulphured.

It is especially important to buy organic dried fruits because chemical sprays are even more concentrated on these.

Raw Materials
For Raw Food Preparation

Vegetables

Leafies
Lettuce
Spinach
Cabbage (red, green)
Napa Cabbage
Chinese Cabbage
Bok Choy
Chard
Collards
Kale

Roots/Stalks
Celery
Carrots
Parsnips
Potatoes (red)
Sweet potatoes
Turnip/Rutabaga
Beets
Jerusalem artichokes
Red radish
Daikon radish
Jicama
Asparagus

Allium family
Garlic
Onions (red, yellow,
    white, sweet)
Green onions/scallions
Leeks

Vegetables (Fruits)
Broccoli
Cauliflower
Bell pepper- red,
    yellow, orange
Green beans
Zucchini
Yellow/summer squash
Peas
Snow Peas
Corn
Cucumber
Winter squashes
Sprouts
Tomato
Avocado
Mushrooms

17

Raw Materials
For Raw Food Preparation

Fresh Herbs

Parsley
Cilantro
Basil
Oregano
Sage
Thyme
Rosemary
Dill

Fresh herbs are preferential to dry. Use approximately three times the amount of fresh when substituting for dried herbs.

Ginger
No need to peel.
Crush with a
garlic press or
store in freezer and
grate as needed

Dried Herbs/Spices

Basil
Cayenne powder
Celery seed
Chili powder
Cinnamon
Cumin, ground
Curry powder
Cloves, ground
Dill weed
Garlic powder
Mustard, seed/ground
Onion powder
Oregano
Paprika
Parsley
Poultry seasoning
Pumpkin pie spice
Rosemary
Sage
Thyme
Turmeric

Raw Materials

For Raw Food Preparation

Nuts

Almonds
Hazelnuts
Brazil nuts
Pecans
Macadamias
Walnuts
Pine nuts
Coconut

Seeds

Sesame seeds
Flax seeds
Chia seeds*
Sunflower seeds
Pumpkin seeds
Sprouting seeds
(clover, radish, broccoli, etc.)

Grains

Sweet brown rice
Quinoa
Buckwheat groats (raw)

Beans/Legumes

Garbanzo beans
Mung beans
Whole dried peas

Note on Grains/Beans

*Personally I am not keen
on recipes made with
raw grains and beans.
I believe they are best
(for several reasons)
in cooked form.*

* Though chia seeds aren't specified in many recipes, they can often be used interchangeably with flax seeds (1/3 the amount of flax specified).

Raw Materials
For Raw Food Preparation

Oils

Olive oil
Coconut oil
Flax oil
Other good oils:
   Sunflower oil
   Hemp oil, etc.
Tahini (raw)
Almond butter (raw)

Thickeners

Psyllium
Flax seed
Chia seed

Flavorings

Peppermint oil/extract
Carob powder (raw)
Cacao powder (raw)
   To substitute cacao powder
   for carob in the recipes, add
   ½ the amount and additional sweetener

Miscellaneous

Unrefined sea salt
Apple cider vinegar
   (raw, unpasteurized)

Raw local honey

Sea vegetables
kelp granules and powder
are interchangeable

Prepared mustard (raw)
This is one of the only
prepared foods I use in
in my recipes. Find one
prepared with raw vinegar
and stoneground mustard

Items followed by (raw)
are ones that can
be difficult to find
in a truly raw form

Essential Basics for Your
Raw Food Pantry

Fresh Produce

Lettuce/Spinach/Greens
Carrots
Celery
Red/sweet onions
Garlic

Tomatoes
Avocados
Oranges
Lemons
Bananas
Apples

Dates
Raisins

Seasonings/Additions

Olive oil
Raw honey
Raw apple cider vinegar
Unrefined sea salt

Sun-dried tomatoes
Carob powder
Psyllium powder

Cinnamon
Basil
Oregano
Onion powder
Garlic powder

Nuts/Seeds

Sunflower seeds
Sesame seeds (tahini)
Flax and/or chia seeds

Almonds
Walnuts/Pecans

Ingredient Information

Special Considerations

Unrefined sea salt   Use unrefined gray or pink sea salt, investigating that it hasn't been heated in processing. Fine ground refined sea salt has usually been heated to 200 degrees for processing.

Cranberries   Because the season of availability is so short, be sure to buy some extra to freeze or dehydrate for future use.

Coconut   Be sure to find unsweetened, unpasteurized coconut shreds or flakes if you are not using fresh coconut (all coconut should be refrigerated).

Sesame seeds   If using unhulled sesame seeds- soak overnight to neutralize some of the oxalic acid in the hulls (then use as is or grind into tahini).

Ingredients I have chosen not to use:

Agar Agar   A sea vegetable used for thickening. It is not raw, but has been boiled in processing.

Nutritional Yeast Powder imparts cheesy flavor to dishes, but has been heated in processing.

Wild Rice has been parched in processing.
   If using: soak 36-48 hours- changing water twice, then drain, rinse and use.

Cashews Even "raw" cashews have been heated to remove them from the shell (substitute with macadamias, pecans or pine nuts).

Young coconuts These appear in many raw food recipes yet since they can be difficult to locate, I've not made them a regular ingredient in any of my recipes. If you can locate them, however, I encourage you to give them a try. First get some instruction on how to open them, then enjoy the meat and milk on their own or try them as a wonderful addition to smoothies.

Ingredients I like to use lots of!

Green vegetables Rich in chlorophyll (only in raw state).
Chlorophyll detoxifies the bloodstream.
Chlorophyll oxygenates the blood and
cells of the body.

A wide variety of vegetables (including cruciferous)-
rich in minerals, pure water and other nutrients.

A wide variety of fruits Easy to digest and rich in
vitamins, antioxidants and pure water.

Regarding Nuts and Seeds

Nuts and seeds are rich in beneficial oils and minerals but should not be over-consumed. A good principle regarding an appropriate amount of nuts/seeds is based on how much you would comfortably shell and enjoy at one sitting. Because they are so high in protein and fat they should make up a smaller amount of our diet than other food categories, so this practical guideline comes in handy. As a rule of thumb, it would probably be best to limit your nut and seed consumption to about a handful (about ½ cup) per day. These can be enjoyed on their own as a snack, with fruit, in a dressing or dip or as part of an entrée or dessert recipe.

In terms of digestibility, it's always best to presoak nuts and seeds before eating or using in a recipe. Nuts and seeds, in their raw state, contain enzyme inhibitors that prevent premature sprouting, but also interfere with proper digestion. Soaking removes the enzyme inhibitors, encouraging easier digestion and better assimilation. See the **Soakables Chart** (pg. 26) for how long to soak each. If you prefer crisp nut, you can dehydrate the nuts following soaking and still get the benefits of the soaking process.

It can be all too easy to eat too many nuts and seeds when you begin on your "raw adventure". They taste great, satisfy the desire for rich food and are incorporated into many tasty dips and desserts. There are certain indicators that you can watch for if you may be overeating protein-dense foods like nuts and seeds:

- Increase in body odor
- Bad gas
- Foods 'sour' the stomach
- Sour-smelling bowel movements

Benefits of Soaking and Sprouting

1. In keeping with nature- birds and small animals carry nuts and seeds in their mouths, cheeks and pouches before eating (to soften and begin germination).
2. Brings nuts, seeds, grains and bean to life- triggers the process of growth. Soaked and sprouted foods aren't just raw- they are truly living foods.
3. Washes away enzyme inhibitors (designed to protect seed but interferes with digestion), phytic acid (inhibits the absorption of calcium, zinc and iron) and oxalic acid (interferes with calcium assimilation) - all factors that can inhibit proper digestion and utilization of nutrients.
4. Makes nuts, seeds, grains and beans easier to chew.
5. Simplifies digestion and improves assimilation of nutrients by changing fats into simple fatty acids, proteins into amino acids and carbohydrates into simple sugars.
6. Increases enzyme and vitamin content of foods.

Flavors, Textures and Characteristics of Soaked Nuts

Macadamias- neutral, oily, crisp
Almonds- sweet, smooth (with skin= grainy)
Brazil nut- warm, earthy, oily, smooth
Hazelnut- warm, earthy, gritty
Pecan- faintly nutty, soft
Walnut- sharper, smooth

Soakables

Nuts

Almonds, Walnuts, Pecans, Macadamias, Brazil nuts, Hazelnuts, Pine nuts, etc.

Seeds

Sunflower, Pumpkin, Sesame, Flax, Chia
- Add to salads
- Use in making dressings, dips, fillings and treats
- Use in dehydrated crackers, cookies and loaves

Dried Fruit

Dates, Raisins, Prunes, Apricots, Sun-dried Tomatoes, etc.
- Use to sweeten sauces, dressings, etc.
- Use in dehydrated cookies, crackers, etc.

Sproutables

Small Seeds

Clover, Radish, Cabbage, Broccoli, etc.
- Add sprouts to salads

Beans

Mung beans, Whole peas, Chickpeas/Garbanzo beans
- Add to salads
- Use in making dips and entrees

Grains

Buckwheat Groats, Sweet Brown Rice, Quinoa
- For making salads, entrees and cereals
- Dehydrated in crackers, cereals, cookies and other treats

Soaking Timetable

Nuts		**Seeds**	
Almonds	8-12 hrs	Sunflower	6-12 hours
Brazil nuts	8-12 hrs	Pumpkin	6-12 hours
Hazelnuts	8-12 hrs	Sesame	6-12 hours
Walnuts	4-12 hrs	Flax	1-2 hours
Pecans	2-4 hours	Chia	1-2 hours
Macadamias	2-4 hours		
Pine nuts	2-4 hour		

Dried Fruits- At least 1 hour

Simplify your soaking: Soak hard nuts overnight.
Soak softs nuts and seeds for a few hours.
When soaking a combination, just soak together overnight.

Sprouting Timetable

All seeds, beans and grains need to be presoaked at least 12 hours (overnight) but preferably for 24 hours before sprouting. Refrigerate if any longer than 8 hours. (Brown rice and chickpeas do well with even 36 hours of soaking.)

Sprout (rinse and drain 2x/day) **for an additional:**
    Small seeds (clover, radish, etc.)
        Start with 1-2 Tbsp., harvest 3-6 days after soaking
    Beans

Mung	½ cup	2-3 days
Whole Peas	1 cup	2-3 days
Chickpeas	1 cup	2-3 days

    Grains

Buckwheat Groats	2 cups	2-3 days
Sweet Brown Rice	2 cups	2-3 days
Quinoa	2 cups	1-2 days

27

Soaking/Sprouting Discussion and Tips

Sprouting can seem a very intimating venture when you see all the sprouting guides and varying instructions and diagrams available. I'm going to make this description as simple and straightforward as possible, making the process as uniform as I can. I want this to strike you as do-able (at least attemptable) because sprouting can be such a gratifying experience *("I'm growing something!")* and provides such a healthful addition to your diet.

There are many containers suitable for soaking and sprouting, but I prefer glass quart canning jars (with wide mouths). They are easy to use when rinsing and draining, you can see the sprouts quite well, and canning jars are just so 'homey' looking! All the suggested amounts of seeds are suited for growth in a 1-quart canning jar.

Before soaking, check over and rinse all seeds, beans and grains. Soak in purified water- add plenty, they may absorb more than you might think. It's okay to use tap water for rinsing thereafter.

You can soak at room temperature for the first 12 hours, then drain, replace water and continue soaking in the refrigerator.

In-between rinses, keep stored at a 45 degree angle (to allow water to continue to drain and air to circulate) in a dark cupboard or drawer (or at least under a dark towel on your counter).

It's easiest to remember to simply rinse upon rising in the morning and before going to bed (It's like brushing your teeth!). On especially warm days, a mid-day rinse might not be a bad idea.

While rinsing, swish sprouts in jar so loose hulls are encouraged to surface and wash away with the rinse water. Removing the hulls helps keep the sprouts stay fresher longer.

Sprout until sprouts are at least as long as the original seed, except for smaller seeds, which sprout for a longer amount of time.

There is controversy about when to eat the sprouts of small seeds. Many suggest eating when two small leaves have appeared and a time in the sun has been allowed for the greening up of those leaves. Some indicate they should be eaten before or after the "two leaf stage" of growth, because the two leaves naturally contain a small amount of toxin that discourages animals from eating the baby plant. Who knows?!

Notes on Sprouting Specific Grains

Quinoa Quinoa naturally has a bitter coating and should be rinsed well before soaking and sprouting to remove it.
Buckwheat Buckwheat develops a gelatinous liquid while soaking. Be sure to rinse well after soaking before using.

Easy Sprouting Instructions

Materials

Quart canning jar

Plastic mesh lid or metal canning ring (or elastic band) to
secure screen or netting to cover jar opening

Process

1. Place seeds in jar and fill jar with purified water.
   Cover with screen. Soak overnight.
2. The next morning (with screen in place) drain off water.
   Rinse by holding under running faucet. Swirl gently, then
   drain. Prop jar at an angle (with screen facing down) in a
   cupboard or drawer (out of sunlight).
3. Until sprouts have reached desired length, rinse and drain
   each morning (upon rising) and each evening (before
   retiring). In the rinsing process, swishing gently will allow
   loosened hulls to rise to top and be rinsed away.
4. Store full-grown sprouts in the refrigerator.

Specifics on Some Simple Sprouts

Clover/Radish Sprouts- *great on salads and as a garnish*
- Begin with 1-2 Tbsp. of seed per quart jar
- Sprout length- 1-2"
- Growing time- 4-5 days
- Place in sun on last day to "green up"

Mung Bean Sprouts- *great on salads and in Asian dishes*
- Begin with ¾ cup mung beans per quart jar
- Sprout length- 2-3"
- Growing time- 3-4 days

Storage of Soaked/Sprouted Foods

Sprouts will keep for up to a week in the refrigerator
Sprouts from **large seeds** can be kept in the refrigerator, covered with water, for many days. (Refresh water every couple of days). Sprouts from **smaller seeds** should be drained and refrigerated. Rinse and drain every few days.

After soaking nuts and seeds for prescribed amount of time, add new purified water and store covered in the refrigerator until ready to use, for up to one week. Change soak water every 2 to 3 days.

Storage of Fermented Foods
(ex.: cultured vegetables, almond cheese)

Because fermented foods are rich in beneficial bacteria, they can be stored in the refrigerator for a long period of time. Nut/seed cheeses can be stored for at least 1-2 weeks and cultured vegetables, when stored in well-sealed containers, can be stored for months in the refrigerator.

Benefits of Fermented Foods

1. Rich in enzymes
2. Digestion has been simplified because the fats have been changed into simple fatty acids, proteins into amino acids and carbohydrates into simple sugars.
3. Helpful in building healthy bacteria in the intestines.

Raw Food Prep Tips

Mottos for wholesome food preparation

"Start Earlier" for wholesome eating
Whole, natural foods generally take longer to cook so you have to begin preparing brown rice or potatoes, for instance, earlier than you would white rice or pasta- but it's really no more work on your part.

"Plan Ahead" for raw eating
Raw food preparation often involves presoaking an ingredient or using a dehydrator, so you often need to think in advance of meal time for certain recipes. I have indicated in the "PREP" section (between the ingredient list and directions for each recipe) any required preparatory work so it won't come as a surprise.   **but. . .**
Plenty of the raw food recipes in this book require no preparatory work *(they're almost instant!)*.

Presoak nuts and seeds in quart canning jars. This way you can easily see what you are soaking and can easily change the water and recap the jar. Quart-size canning jars also usually have cup measures on the side that simplify the measuring of your ingredients.

More often than not, when you **process with a heavy duty blender**, you'll find it most helpful to keep the plunger in place to help push down and circulate the ingredients. The cap for the lid is less frequently used (for dressings, etc.).

When using a heavy-duty blender for raw food prep that requires a very smooth texture, be sure to have about **4 cups of ingredients** in the blender so it can easily circulate with aid of the plunger.

Some ingredients are listed by number or portion

For example: 2 carrots, ¼ sweet onion, ½ red pepper

Understandably, sizes of items vary, so use your own good judgment in determining amounts.

Remember- the amounts recommended in these recipes were arrived at by trial and error. Your experimentation may lead you to an even better recipe!

Sweet and red onions are recommended in the recipes
Personally I find that traditional onions (yellow, white) are too strong in raw food recipes. Many people can tolerate and even enjoy them- so I encourage you to explore if they work for you. My recipes recommend sweet onions (like Vidalias) or red onions because they are milder. Often a recipe asks for ½ or ¼ of an onion. Here you'll need to use your judgment. I find that those fractions correlate pretty well to cup sizes (½ onion is about ½ cup of onion).

Presoaked nuts, seeds, and beans can be frozen until needed for use in a recipe.

When you've made a **large quantity of nut loaves or burgers**, freeze any excess for later use.

When you have **excess dips or fillings**, you can spread them thinly onto parchment paper and dehydrate into crackers or for use as a crumbled topping for salads. No opportunity to use that **extra salsa**? Mix it with soaked flax seeds and dehydrate into crackers!

To speed the ripening of avocados and other fruit (pears, peaches, bananas, etc.) put in a brown paper bag in a warm place. Ripe avocados can be refrigerated until ready to use (store unused half with pit in place).

Dressings, dips and sauces that have been **made with fresh lemon juice** will keep quite well. Salsa and dressing can be kept for up to two weeks as the lemon helps keeps it fresh.

Make your own shredded coconut: Find the soft eye at the end of coconut (one of the three). Open hole with knife, screwdriver, etc. Shake out coconut milk *(Enjoy!).* Put coconut in a canvas bag, then 'whack' repeatedly on a hard surface (outdoor patio, sidewalk, driveway), until the coconut has broken up adequately. Bring inside and separate the coconut shell from the meat. Rinse the meat off in a colander. Peel the outer brown skin off the meat with a vegetable peeler. Process small pieces of the coconut in a food processor until it has shredded to the desired fineness. Use right away or put in freezer for later use.

To ensure garlic is finely minced for a recipe, add it on its own to a food processor and continue running the processor until the garlic has been reduced to small pieces, thrown to the sides of the container.

To thicken or firm-up a dish, add:

Flax- gelatinous- good for thickening liquids or for binding ingredients (like in dehydrated crackers)

Chia- similar to flax (use 1/3 of amount specified for flax)

Psyllium- firm- good for firming up more solid dishes, especially those that will be refrigerated before serving (like pies).

Keep On Hand for Quick and Easy Prep of Raw Meals

A little planning/preparing ahead can take you far! Try not to get caught without having something quick and easy available to eat- otherwise it becomes too tempting to make a poor choice.

Frozen bananas for smoothies and soft-serve ice-cream

Frozen berries and fruit for adding to smoothies

Presoaked almonds (keep refrigerated for up to a week)
Soak almonds for at least 8 hours, rinse and add fresh water every couple of days.
1 cup dry almonds= about 1 $^2/_3$ cup soaked almonds

Prepared tahini- ready for use in future recipes.

Keep a **small jar of soaked sun-dried tomatoes** in the refrigerator for use in dressings, dips, dehydrates, etc.

A batch of homemade **mayonnaise** has many uses and applications and is great to keep on hand.

Make dressings in double or triple batches so you have more than enough for a week. Extra amounts can be frozen for later use.

Make **bulk supplies of dips, fillings and sauces** like hummus, seed-based dips, mayonnaise, salsa, etc. Keep some on hand in the refrigerator, then freeze extra in handy portions.

Make a **large portion of Marinara Sauce** (pg. 102) and freeze in portions in glass bowls or resealable freezer baggies for quick pasta nights (place sealed baggie in a bowl of warm water to defrost and warm for use).

Marinated greens get more tender and flavorful with time. It's not a bad idea to make up a batch weekly to add to a meal as desired.

The taste, texture and digestibility of most nuts are greatly improved by soaking. Go ahead and **soak and dehydrate a variety of nuts** before you have plans for them. The dehydrated nuts can be stored in glass jars in your pantry, refrigerator or freezer.

Every few weeks prepare **a variety of dehydrates** to keep on hand- crackers, chips, cookies, fruit leathers, etc.

General Eating Tips

1. Consider adding fresh vegetable juices to your diet- a concentrated source of nutrition that simultaneously builds and cleanses the body.
2. 1 Tbsp. of ground flax in a glass of water once or twice a day serves as a great fiber supplement.
3. Aim for a raw fruit meal for breakfast or lunch.
4. Eat fruit separate from other foods, as a snack or meal (less of an issue if eating an all-raw diet).
   Some people find nuts/seeds combine well with fruits.
5. Regularly begin largest meal of the day with a big salad.
6. Chew slowly and thoroughly.
7. Drink water at least ten minutes before or one hour after meals.
8. Watch that you take in enough liquids each day.
   Your urine should be almost colorless and odorless.
   Fresh juices and produce are the best source. Rehydrate in the morning with a pint or so of water upon rising. Take water with you when you leave home.

Keep It Simple

Though there are a great variety of recipes offered in this book, I want to encourage you to keep things simple by planning your meals around easy, tried-and true-favorites, and then incorporate those foods that are richer or require more preparation now and again or for special occasions.

Raw eating can be quite simple:
Morning- fresh vegetable or fruit **juices**
Light meal- **fruit meal**- whole fruits, fruit salad, smoothies
Large meal- **large salad served with** a dip or filling-based dish, flax crackers, or less frequently, a pasta or loaf.

Raw Meal Ideas

Breakfast
Vegetable juices
Fruit juices
Fruit recipes

Light Meal
Fruit recipes
Salad recipes
Veggies and Dips/Fillings
Soups with Dehydrated Crackers

Snacks
Fruit recipes
Veggies and Dips/Fillings
Dehydrated Snacks
Desserts/Treats

Large Meal
Large salad or marinated greens
Accompanied by an entrée:
Veggies and Dips/Fillings
Stuffed vegetables
Soups with Dehydrated Crackers
Nutmeat dishes
Veggie pasta and sauce
Cereals (soaked or dehydrated)
Dessert entrees

Raw Basics

The following recipes have wide appeal and make up the majority of our meals, so considering trying these soon! They are great for beginners, and will quickly become basics in your raw foods repertoire.

Fruit salads
Fruit smoothies
Vegetable salads
Veggies with dips or fillings
Flax crackers
Fruit-and-nut truffles
Soft-serve ice cream

In the index of each section of the cookbook,
I've put in **bold** those recipes that are basics, staples or
just plain favorites in our home.
You may want to begin your "raw adventure"
by trying some of these recipes first.

Homemade Basic Ingredients

Some recipes call for mayonnaise, tahini, salsa or other ingredients that you can (and will probably need to) make from scratch. Recipes for these basic ingredients are located in this book and the page numbers for them are usually indicated.

"PREP" notes - for recipes that require some advance preparation

I have included a "PREP" section following the ingredient list for those recipes that have nuts, seeds, grains or other ingredients that need to be soaked or sprouted prior to assembling the dish.

Note: If you keep presoaked almonds on hand, many of the recipes don't require a day's advance preparation.

Recipe Sections

Juices

There are many good books on juicing, so I won't take much space here to discuss it, yet the benefits of consuming fresh juices must be at least touched upon.

Consuming the freshly extracted juices of fruits and vegetables is the most efficient and effective way to get dense nutrition to your body. Where supplements miss the mark (isolated nutrients in questionable ratios from even more questionable sources), juicing is the best way to get real nutrition from whole food sources into your system. Only the fiber has been removed, so all the nutrients remain in their natural ratios, with all the accompanying enzymes and other aids needed for their assimilation.

Juices are best consumed on an empty stomach, at least half an hour before eating any other foods. The benefit of drinking freshly extracted juices is based in the fact that the fiber has been removed, so digestion is more efficient and more nutrients are assimilated. If you drink juice with solid foods you are defeating a significant portion of this benefit.

The basic recipe on the following page will produce between five to seven 8-ounce glasses of juice.

Our Basic Juice Recipe

For every five-pound bag of carrots (ideally, organic juicing carrots)

Add   1-2 Granny Smith apples
        and any combination of beets, celery, cucumber,
            parsley, spinach, kale, chard, collards, beet greens,
            romaine lettuce, ginger, etc.

Make enough juice for the whole day (or for two days, depending upon the quality of your juicer).   Strain into 8-ounce canning jars, lid tightly, then store in refrigerator or pack in an insulated bag with an ice pack for taking with you.

Be sure to use a masticating juicer to preserve the nutrients and enzymes. Masticating juicers can cost more than centrifugal juicers, but the price difference is quickly made up for in juice quantity and quality.

There is a world of great tasting and health-promoting juices at your fingertips when you make your own fresh juices. I encourage you to get a book on juicing and begin exploring some tasty combinations!

Fruit Recipes

Fruit Recipes

Check for many more fruit-based recipes in the
Snacks/Dehydrates and **Desserts/Treats** sections.

Whole Fruits

Oranges

Grapefruit

Kiwi

Pineapple

Mango

Papaya

Grapes

Strawberries

Blueberries

Raspberries

Apples

Pears

Peaches

Plums

Bananas

Melons, etc.

Any of these fruits on their own or in combination with others, make a very pleasant breakfast, lunch, snack or light dinner.

(For ideal food combining, sour fruits and sweet fruits should be eaten separately.) Citrus fruits, kiwis and berries are good together. Bananas with grapes is nice.

Melons should always be eaten on their own because they digest so quickly.

Fruit Salad

Cut any variety of the following fresh fruit into chunks
(as well as any other favorites) and serve combined in a bowl

apples	*mango*
pears	*papaya*
peaches	*blueberries*
nectarines	*raspberries*
plums	*strawberries*
bananas	*pineapple*
grapes	*oranges*

Some recommended combinations:

Papaya, mango, pineapple (with or without banana)

Pear, apple, date and pecan

Kiwi, strawberry, apple, banana, blueberries

Apple, pear, banana, dates

Banana, orange, grapes, pecans

Any of these combinations are nice topped with chopped nuts
or with a **Fruit Salad Cream** or **Sauce** (pg. 48).

Fruit Salad Cream

$^1/_3$ cup almonds or pecans

½ cup water

juice of 1 orange

1 frozen banana

1 Tbsp. flax oil

1 Tbsp. honey (or 3 dates)

PREP: Presoak nuts (almonds- 8 hours, pecans- 2 hours)

Process nuts, juice and water in blender until smooth. Add rest of ingredients and whip until smooth.

Optional: replace orange juice with another ½ cup of water

Serve over berries, cut peaches or a fruit salad.

Fruit Salad Sauce

Juice of 2 oranges

Juice of ½ of lemon

 (more or less based on taste)

$^1/_3$ cup dates, pitted

4-6 strawberries or

 ½ cup of other berries

Process all ingredients in blender until smooth. Serve over a fruit salad.

Fruit Kabobs

Apple   Pears

Kiwi   Peaches

Grapes   Strawberries

Pineapple   Mango

Alternate fruit on skewer.

Very pleasing to the eye and palate.
Basically a fruit salad on a stick!

Melon Bowl

Wash the outside of the melon well before cutting (any bacteria on the skin is introduced to the inside as it is cut). Cut melon in half, scoop out seeds and serve as is.

- or -

Cut open a couple of different kinds of melons. Scoop or slice into bite-size pieces and serve in bowls.

Note on proper food combining- *always eat melons on their own. They digest more quickly than other fruit and can cause problems when eaten with them.*

Ambrosia

4 oranges $^2/_3$ cup walnuts or pecans
2 cups chopped pineapple $^1/_3$ cup shredded coconut

Cut oranges into 8 wedges with serrated knife. Remove any seeds, then cut away from rind and into pieces. Mix all ingredients together and chill until ready to serve.

Variation: Use a variety of oranges, tangerines and other citrus fruits instead of just oranges, if you'd like.

Waldorf Salad

3 apples, diced   ½+ cup mayonnaise*
3 celery ribs, chopped   2 tsp. lemon juice/vinegar
1 cup walnuts, chopped   ¼ tsp. cinnamon
1 ½ cups halved grapes   opt: ½ cup raisins

Mix ingredients in right column. Combine in a bowl with the ingredients in the left column. Serve chilled.

* almond-based mayonnaise recipe on page 100

Variation: Add the juice of 1 orange in place of lemon juice

Berries with Whipped Topping

strawberries, raspberries, blueberries, etc.

Place whole, sliced or chopped berries in a bowl. Top with **Whipped Topping** (recipe below). If desired, sprinkle with chopped nuts.

Variation: Combine cut bananas with berries before adding whipped topping.

Whipped Topping

¹/₃ cup soaked almonds   *1 Tbsp. flax oil*

1 cup water   *4-6 strawberries*

1 ½ frozen banana   *1 Tbsp. honey, to taste*

Whip ingredients together in blender. Serve immediately.

Peaches and Cream

6 peaches or nectarines   1- 1 ½ cup water
$^1/_3$ cup pecans   pinch of sea salt
2 frozen bananas   opt: 1 Tbsp. flax oil

PREP: Presoak pecans for at least 2 hours.

Cut peaches or nectarines in slices or pieces. Process rest of ingredients in a blender until smooth. Serve peaches or nectarines in bowls and then top with prepared "cream".

Creamy Pudding

1 avocado   1 frozen banana
2 bananas   4 dates, presoaked

Whip together all ingredients in blender and serve. Try sprinkling with chopped nuts or coconut, or add ¼ cup carob (or 2 Tbsp. cacao) powder to make a chocolate version.
Note: Be sure to use **very ripe** avocados and bananas.

"Try it, you'll like it."
You might be surprised by how good this is!

Applesauce

2-4 organic apples   *opt: ½ tsp. cinnamon*
1-2 tsp. lemon juice

Wash and core apples (peel commercial ones). Cut into large chunks. Puree in blender with lemon juice (and cinnamon).

Variations: Add a few strawberries or cranberries before pureeing. Or add ½ cup raisins after pureeing apples and allow to sit for a short while so the raisins have time to plump up before serving (or presoak raisins).

Apple Gelatin

3 apples   *2 tsp. psyllium powder*
2 tsp. lemon juice   *opt: berries, pears, etc.*

Wash and core apples. Puree with lemon juice (and any optional fruits) in blender. Mix in psyllium powder. Allow to sit in blender for a few minutes, then mix again. Pour into a small bowl and refrigerate to gel.

Variation: Add cut up bananas, grapes, pineapple, etc. to pureed mixture before gelling.

Fruit Yogurt

¾ cup sunflower seeds   1 banana

juice of 1 lemon   1 cup (frozen) fruit

²/₃ cup water   pinch of sea salt

Process sunflower seeds, lemon juice, sea salt and water till smooth in a blender. Add banana and fruit, and then process until smooth once more.

Frozen fruit could include strawberries, raspberries, blueberries, peaches, mangos, etc.

Fruit Jelly/Jam/Gelatin

1-1½ cups of fruit (strawberries, blueberries, or 2 apples)

1-2 Tbsp. honey   2-3 tsp. psyllium powder

2 tsp. lemon juice

Process ingredients in food processor, until smooth (add honey and lemon to taste). Refrigerate to gel. Combine fruits for a mixed fruit jelly or jam (for ex: apple strawberry).

This can be served spread on other foods (sweet crackers or cookies). But there's no reason the kids (or grown-ups) can't eat it as is- it's a very wholesome fruit gelatin.

Dried Fruits

Be sure to find organic, unsulphured, unsweetened dried fruit

raisins	*figs*
prunes	*dates*
apricots	*papaya*
apples	*mango, etc.*

Ideally, rinse dried fruit with boiling water to wash away any molds, mildew, or bacteria. Presoak if using in a recipe that requires plump, juicy fruit. Store rinsed (and soaked) dried fruit in refrigerator if not consuming right away.

Dried fruits are great on their own or
combined with nuts or seeds as a snack.

Trail Mix

almonds	*raisins*
walnuts	*dates*
sunflower seeds	*other dried fruit*
pumpkin seeds	*(apples, figs, dates, etc.)*

Mix together any combination in any ratio (using more of your favorite nuts and fruit!) and store in a container.

Great for taking on trips.

Fruit with Nut Butter

Sliced apples
Sliced bananas

Spread fruit slices with raw almond butter, pumpkin seed butter or other raw nut butter.

Variation: Mix nut butter with a small amount of honey or carob powder before spreading on fruit.

Celery sticks can also be stuffed with nut butters.

Stuffed Dates

dates
almonds, walnuts or pecans

Slit date open lengthwise and remove pit. Replace pit with whole nuts.

Optional: Stuff dates with nut butter, or nut butter mixed with carob powder or honey, before topping with a nut.

*These are nice arranged attractively on a platter
and served at the holidays.*

Preparing Oranges *for fruit salads or smoothies*

The simplest way I've found to prepare oranges is to cut the orange lengthwise into 8 wedges with a serrated knife. Cut away any easily accessible tough membrane and remove seeds from each wedge, before cutting from skin and adding to a salad or the blender.

Freezing Bananas

Frozen bananas are the base for smoothies, banana milk and other treats (like creamy pudding and soft-serve ice cream). When bananas are heavily speckled (even all brown), they are in the perfect state for peeling and freezing. Keep a stash of them on hand in a glass container or resealable freezer bags in the freezer. Stock up when you see these "overripe" bananas on clearance shelves in the produce section.

Freezing Other Fruit

Stock up on and freeze peaches, strawberries, blueberries, grapes, etc., as they come into season and are a good buy.

Fruit Smoothies

These can be a great part of any day-
for breakfast or lunch, or as an afternoon or evening snack
Use your creativity with this great fruit staple!

2 oranges*
2 handfuls of blueberries,
   strawberries, pineapple,
   mango or other fruit you
   may have on hand**

$^1/_3$ cup nuts***
½ cup water or ice
1-2 Tbsp. flax oil
2 frozen bananas
opt: 1 apple (cored)

Peel, cut and add fruits to the blender. Add rest of ingredients and puree until smooth. *Puree the oranges, nuts, water and any 'seedy' berries before adding the other ingredients, to ensure they're thoroughly processed.*
* or one cup of orange juice (ideally, fresh squeezed).
** about 1 ½ cups of fruit. I tend to use frozen berries.
*** walnuts, almonds, pecans, etc.- ideally presoaked
Using **fresh bananas** instead of frozen? Add some ice in place of some of the liquid for a better consistency.

Great served topped with chopped nuts (almonds, walnuts, pecans), shredded coconut and/or ground flax.

Green Smoothie   For a great nutritional boost- add spinach, kale, chard or other greens to the blender.

Fruit Soup

You have complete freedom and flexibility when it comes to making a blend of fruits into a smoothie. We've enjoyed thousands with an incredible variety of fruits.

Our favorite variation of a fruit smoothie is what we call fruit "soup". We often have fruit soup for lunch. It's something like a cross between a smoothie (drinkable) and sorbet (ice-cream consistency)- and we eat it in a bowl with toppings. Sometimes we have it with chopped fresh fruit (like strawberries, mangos, raspberries, etc.) and chopped nuts (walnuts, pecans, almonds) and almost always with freshly ground flax seed (ground flax is similar to toasted wheat germ but raw and nutritionally superior).

We base our fruit soup on whatever fresh and frozen fruit we have on hand, but it usually includes oranges, apples, blueberries (or mangos and strawberries) plus bananas, nuts, flax oil and just a small amount of water added for blend-ability. Served in bowls, it makes a quick, easy and incredibly tasty lunch.

Fruit Smoothie Combinations

Pina Colada Smoothie

2 cups pineapple

4 frozen bananas

4 oranges

½ cup coconut

Strawberry Mango Smoothie

1 mango

1 pint strawberries

3 oranges

4-5 frozen bananas

Creamy Orange Smoothie

4 oranges

10 presoaked almonds

3 frozen bananas

$^2/_3$ cup water or ice

Banana Mango Sorbet

2 oranges   4-5 frozen bananas
1 mango   1-2 Tbsp. flax oil
$^1/_3$ cup water

Process in blender until smooth, but still firm. (Freeze the mango ahead for a very thick sorbet).

Optional toppings: *Chopped strawberries*
Chopped almonds, pecans, etc.

Banana-sicles

Cut bananas in half and poke a popsicle stick into each half. Roll in **Carob Sauce** (pg. 217) and freeze in a glass containers or resealable freezer bags.

Optional: After coating in **Carob Sauce**, roll the frozen banana in chopped nuts and/or coconut before freezing.

Salads

Salads

Green Salad Components

*Keep a variety of salad components on hand
so your salads remain interesting and varied.*

The salad base- *any combination of:*

> green leaf, red leaf or romaine lettuce
>
> spinach leaves
>
> small pieces of kale, or other "exotic" greens
>
> thinly sliced green or red cabbage

Some of the usual toppings

carrot, grated or sliced	red/sweet onion
cucumbers	tomatoes
red or yellow peppers	celery
	radishes

Toppings that add a little more interest

zucchini	sprouts
cauliflower	summer squash
broccoli florets	beets, grated
green peas	avocado
marinated tomatoes	herbs- parsley,
marinated vegetables	basil, cilantro, etc.

Some even more exceptional toppings

snow peas	*jicama*
broccoli stalks, diced	*kohlrabi*
corn from cob	*fennel*
green onions	*Jerusalem artichokes*
daikon radish	*turnip/rutabaga*
dried fruit	*fresh berries*

Crunchy, flavorful and nutritional additions

nuts *- almonds, walnuts, pecans, pine nuts, etc.*

seeds *- sunflower, pumpkin, sesame, hemp, etc.*

ground flax seed

good oils *- unrefined flax oil, hemp oil, blends, etc.*

. . . **and dressing**, of course!

*When you **make your own dressings** with wholesome,*
raw ingredients and healthful unrefined oils,
you don't need to be as cautious about
the amount of dressing you use.
Just some of the peace of mind that comes with
preparing your own foods!

Salad-Making Tips

Salad spinners and a food processor can be really handy and simplify salad-making. Every day or two we **wash our greens** and spin dry in a salad spinner. We leave the lettuce leaves whole in a covered glass bowl in the refrigerator until we are ready to use them. Then we only break up (or cut) the amount of lettuce that we will be using for that one meal.

We cut, slice, or grate our **salad toppings**, then **add them**
- either directly to our salad plates (full-size dinner plates-who can fit a decent-sized salad in a salad bowl?!)
- or to bowls that will be set at the table from which individuals can create their own salads (salad bar-style).

Each salad is usually sprinkled with **ground flax** and often with some **seeds or nuts**, and topped with homemade **dressing.**

Our salad is always our first course, and usually doesn't leave too much room for what follows!

If you get tired of green salads, be sure to alternate them with some grated salads, coleslaw, a marinated salad, or cut veggies and dip.

Seed-based Salad Toppings

Sunflower Seeds and Pumpkin Seeds

Use whole or grind briefly in a coffee grinder, blender or food processor. Sea vegetables, like nori and dulse, can be added to the seeds before grinding.

Ground pumpkin seeds, paired with a Caesar dressing, make a great parmesan substitute!

Ground Flax

Grind fresh flax (stored in refrigerator or freezer) in a coffee grinder or blender. Grind briefly, to prevent beneficial oils from becoming heated. Use immediately or store in a glass container (a glass canning jar works well) in the refrigerator or freezer. Sprinkle over salads, fruit smoothies or cereal.

Sesame Salt

Process 1 cup of sesame seeds in blender with ½ tsp. sea salt until well ground. Store in refrigerator in glass container and sprinkle over salads or prepared dishes.

Spinach Salad with Simple Dressing

3 Tbsp. olive oil

2 Tbsp. apple cider vinegar

1 Tbsp. honey

¼ sweet onion, chopped

1 garlic clove, crushed

½ tsp. sea salt

large bunch of spinach

1 avocado, sliced

$^1/_3$ cup pine nuts, walnuts,
   or chopped almonds

opt: cherry tomatoes,
   oil-cured olives, red onion

PREP: Combine ingredients in left column and allow to marinate together for at least for one hour.

Break up spinach and serve on plates topped with avocado, nuts and optional toppings. Drizzle with dressing.

Caesar Salad

Romaine lettuce

¼ cup pumpkin seeds

any other salad toppings
that you might like

Break up romaine lettuce leaves. Grind pumpkin seeds in a coffee grinder or food processor, toss with lettuce, then top with either **Garlic Caesar Dressing** (pg. 89) or **Creamy Caesar Dressing** (pg. 90).

Grated Rainbow Salad

beets	red cabbage
carrots	tomatoes slices
summer squash	corn off the cob
zucchini	sliced radishes

Grate beets, carrots, summer squash, zucchini and cabbage, then arrange in concentric rings on a plate or platter. Arrange sliced radishes and tomatoes decoratively in the center or around border, then sprinkle with corn kernels. Individuals can serve onto beds of lettuce and drizzle with dressing.

A nice alternative to the usual green salad.

Simple Cabbage Salad

½ head green cabbage	¼ cup olive oil
½ head red cabbage	½ tsp. garlic powder
1 carrot, grated	½ tsp. sea salt
¼ cup apple cider vinegar	opt: 3 green onions

Shred cabbage. Combine vinegar, oil, garlic powder and sea salt in bowl, then mix in rest of ingredients. Best if allowed to chill at least 1 hour in refrigerator before serving.

Basic Coleslaw

½ head cabbage,   2-3 carrots, grated
    grated or thinly sliced

Mix vegetables (and any other additions) with dressing. Refrigerate for at least one hour before serving.

Basic Coleslaw Dressing

½ cup mayonnaise (pg. 100)   ¼ tsp. sea salt
2 tsp. apple cider vinegar   ¼ tsp. cinnamon
    or lemon juice

Mix with vegetables for basic coleslaw.   -or-

Add ingredients for the two following versions.

Apple Raisin Coleslaw

My favorite. Add: ¾ cup raisins
1 chopped apple   ¼ tsp. cinnamon

Curried Coleslaw

Eliminate cinnamon and add: Sliced red pepper
1-2 tsp. prepared mustard   Diced red onion
½ tsp. curry powder   pinch of cayenne

Caesar Coleslaw

In place of basic slaw dressing, use **Garlic Caesar** (pg. 89) or **Creamy Caesar Dressing** (pg. 90) over the grated vegetables. Add a fresh diced tomato, if desired.

Easy Coleslaw

In place of basic slaw dressing, add **Italian Dressing** (pg. 89) to grated vegetables.

**All slaws can be sprinkled
with nuts or seeds before serving.**

Veggie Slaw

carrot	*broccoli stalks*
turnip	*kohlrabi*
red cabbage	*butternut squash*

Grate veggies and mix with **Coleslaw** dressing (pg. 70).

Turnip, kohlrabi and carrot version

Add 1 tsp. dill weed to basic coleslaw dressing

Butternut squash, red cabbage and raisin version

Add extra cinnamon to basic coleslaw dressing

71

Creamy Coleslaw

2-3 Tbsp. tahini (pg. 100)	½ tsp. paprika
1 Tbsp. apple cider vinegar	½ tsp. ground mustard
3 Tbsp. lemon juice	¼ tsp. ground cumin
1 Tbsp. honey or 4 dates	½+ tsp. sea salt
3 Tbsp. olive/flax oil	1 head cabbage, grated
1/3+ cup water	2 carrots, grated
¼ cup almonds	¾ cup raisins, soaked

PREP: Presoak almonds for at least 8 hours. Sunflower seeds can be substituted for almonds (soak at least 6 hours).

Process all ingredients, except for cabbage, carrots and raisins, in a blender until smooth. Pour over grated vegetables and raisins. Mix well. Serve immediately or store in refrigerator.

Beet and Carrot Salad

3 - 4 beets	2 carrots	juice of 1 lemon

Finely grate beets and carrots. Mix with lemon juice. Chill.

Sounds almost too simple,
but this salad is beautiful and tastes like berries!

Carrot and Raisin Salad

1 lb. carrots (about 8)   ¼ tsp. cinnamon

½ cup raisins   ½ tsp. lemon juice

$^1/_3$ cup mayonnaise (pg. 100)   or apple cider vinegar

2 tsp. honey   opt: 1 chopped apple

Combine wet ingredients and cinnamon. Peel and grate carrots then mix with other ingredients. Refrigerate before serving.

Optional Tahini Dressing

3 Tbsp. tahini (pg. 100)   2 Tbsp. lemon juice

2 Tbsp. flax oil   ¼ tsp. cinnamon

2 Tbsp. water

Stir together and mix with grated carrots and raisins. Serve immediately.

Optional Apple Dressing

½ cup presoaked almonds   1 apple

1 -2 chopped carrots   ¼ tsp. cinnamon

Puree all ingredients and then mix with grated carrots and raisins. Serve immediately.

Raw Cultured Vegetables

(not to be mistaken with store-bought sauerkraut)

Cultured vegetables have a long history in many cultures. Cultured vegetables are simply ground vegetables (primarily cabbage) held in a warm (60-70 degrees), sanitary environment for a few days during which time the friendly bacteria present in the vegetables naturally proliferates. They have a tangy flavor that may take some getting used to. We enjoy ours served on grated carrots and sprouts, topped with good oils and a creamy dressing (to mellow the tanginess).

The benefits of cultured vegetables:
- An excellent source of friendly bacteria.
    Cheaper than probiotic supplements!
- They are "predigested" and easier to assimilate.
    Gentle on a strained digestive system.
- They are very alkaline and cleansing.
    Expect some gas initially (*Sorry.*)

**Cabbage serves as the base for cultured veggies.
Optional additions include:**

Carrots	*Sea vegetables*
Beets	*Garlic*
Celery	*Ginger*
Lemon juice	*Sea salt*
Herbs	

This recipe may look long, but it is not incredibly difficult. It makes a good quantity and keeps well in the refrigerator for 5 months or more in sealed jars.

Simple Cultured Vegetable Recipe

1. Start with a very clean environment and very fresh, organic vegetables.

2. Cabbage is the base- green or red (optional additions are listed on the page to the left). Begin with several heads of cabbage (at least 3). You want to generate a quantity worth the effort of making this recipe.

3. Peel off dry, damaged outer leaves. Peel off several good leaves and reserve aside.

4. **Either:** Grind up the cabbage (and other additions) in a food processor and then beat in a stainless steel pot with a heavy blunt object until the natural juices are released.

> **Or:** (the easier option) Process them through a juicer with the blank attachment in place. In this case you won't need to pound the vegetables after grinding.

5. Fill a large stainless steel pot or glass or ceramic crock about ¾ full with the ground vegetables.

6. Cover well with the reserved cabbage leaves.

7. Press down on leaves, gently but firmly, to compact mixture. Be sure there are no air pockets and veggies are all beneath liquid. Cover the leaves with a large overturned dinner plate- covering as much of the opening of the pot as possible. Fill a couple of canning jars with water and place on the plate to weigh it down.

8. Cover the pot with a clean dishtowel and set in an undisturbed place at room temperature (between 60-70 degrees) for five to seven days. Hot climates and hot seasons are not conducive to making cultured vegetables because the fermentation happens too quickly.

9. After 5-7 days, uncover pot, remove cabbage leaves and wipe away any moldy or discolored vegetables or sections (I usually spoon away discolored vegetables, and wipe the sides of the pot with a paper towel).

10. Pack the cultured vegetables into glass canning jars, seal tightly with lids and refrigerate.

Oriental-Style Napa Salad

½ cup apricots

3 Tbsp. tahini (pg. 100)

1 Tbsp. fresh ginger

1 tsp. prepared mustard

2 Tbsp. apple cider vinegar

3 Tbsp. olive oil

½ tsp. sea salt

$^1/_3$ cup water

1 head Napa cabbage

2 carrots, julienne

½ red pepper, sliced

4 green onions, sliced

2 Tbsp. sesame seeds

PREP: Rinse apricots with boiling water, then briefly soak in purified water.

Process all ingredients in left column with water at top of right column in a blender until smooth. Chop head of Napa cabbage and combine in bowl with carrots, red pepper and green onions. Pour sauce from blender over vegetables and mix together. Sprinkle top with sesame seeds.

Oriental-Style Broccoli Salad

1 head broccoli   ¼ red/sweet onion
2 Tbsp. sesame seeds   or 4 green onions
Sauce ingredients from **Oriental-Style Napa Salad** (pg. 76)

Chop broccoli into fairly large pieces. Chop onion (or green onions) fairly fine.   Prepare sauce and mix with veggies. Sprinkle salad with sesame seeds before serving.

Ginger Napa Cabbage Salad

1 small Napa cabbage-or-   1 head bok choy
½ red pepper slivered   -or-   2 carrots, grated
4 green onions   -or-   ½ sweet onion
2 garlic cloves, crushed   1 tsp. prepared mustard
$^1/_3$ cup apple cider vinegar   1-2 Tbsp. fresh ginger
2 Tbsp. olive oil   (or ½ tsp. ground)
½ tsp. sea salt   pinch cayenne

Chop Napa cabbage or bok choy into 1" strips. Combine together garlic, minced ginger, salt, mustard, vinegar, and cayenne.   Pour over vegetables and mix well. Refrigerate for at least one hour before serving.

Marinades and Marinating Vegetables

Marinades are usually a combination of lemon juice, olive oil, and sea salt with some other optional additions. They are used to preflavor an ingredient before adding to a salad or dish, to tenderize tough vegetables and to mellow the bitterness, intensity or "rawness" of certain vegetables.

Mellowing/Tenderizing Marinade

juice of 1 lemon
2 Tbsp. olive oil
opt: 1 garlic clove, crushed

½ tsp. sea salt
opt: herbs, spices

This is great to use with tough greens (chard, collards, kale, etc.) or firm veggies (broccoli, cauliflower, etc.) to encourage them to tenderize and mellow before serving or using in the preparation of another dish. If you work the marinade into the greens (massage with your hands) it will help tenderize the greens and deepen the flavor. Also great for mellowing the strength of onions- just slice and marinate.

Option: Whole green leaves that have been tenderized can be filled with dips or fillings and rolled into "cabbage rolls".

Marinated Spinach

1 bunch spinach

1 garlic clove

½ tsp. sea salt

juice of 1 lemon

2 Tbsp. olive oil

opt: 1 tomato,
    slice of red onion

Process garlic in food processor, then add salt, lemon, oil (and any optional ingredients you have chosen). Chop spinach and combine in a bowl with marinade. Mix well (helps to gently knead with hands). Let sit at least one hour (up to two days) before serving.

Variation: For a creamier consistency, add a small amount of mayonnaise (pg. 100) to the marinade blend.

Marinated Greens

Choice of a bunch of kale, collards, or chard
2 tomatoes, chopped
Mellowing Marinade *ingredients (pg. 78)*

Trim off center stalks of greens. Roll and slice then chop. Add chopped tomatoes and **Mellowing Marinade** (pg. 78), including garlic clove. Allow to marinate for at least 3-4 hours (preferably overnight) before serving.

Creamy Marinated Greens

Follow directions for **Marinated Greens** (above) except add the following to the marinade before mixing with greens:

2 dates, pitted   *2 tsp. ground cumin*
½ tsp. turmeric   *opt: pinch cayenne*

Marinated Eggplant

juice of 1 lemon

1 Tbsp. oil

1 garlic clove, crushed

½ tsp. sea salt

2 tsp. dried basil

1 eggplant

Thinly slice eggplant then cut crosswise into strips and place in shallow bowl (preferably one that has a lid). Combine the rest of the ingredients above into a marinade and then pour over the eggplant. Allow to marinate at room temperature for a few hours (or longer in the refrigerator). Occasionally stir (or shake, if you have a lidded bowl). Drain off liquid when done marinating.

Serve on salads or with an entrée.

Marinated Eggplant Chips

A dehydrated recipe using same ingredients as above

Slice eggplant into ¼ inch thick rounds. Marinate with mixture above for at least 2-4 hours. Place slices on dehydrating trays and dehydrate for at least 8 hours at 100 degrees, until crisp.

Marinated Veggie Salad

1 bunch broccoli florets   2 carrots, thinly sliced

½ head cauliflower   ½ red onion, thinly sliced

$^1/_3$ cup **Italian dressing** -or- optional dressing (below)

Break or cut broccoli and cauliflower into bite-sized pieces. Combine with other veggies in a bowl. Pour dressing over top. Mix well and allow to chill for several hours before serving (stirring on occasion).

Optional additions:

 1 red pepper, sliced or chopped

 1 tomato, chopped or sliced

 1 avocado, chopped and added before serving

Optional Dressing for Marinated Vegetables:

juice of 1 lemon   ¼ cup chopped parsley

2 tsp. apple cider vinegar ¼ tsp. garlic powder

$^1/_3$ cup olive oil   ¼ tsp. basil and oregano

2 Tbsp. chives   ¼ tsp. sea salt

Mix all ingredients together and combine with vegetables.

Marinated Tomatoes

2 tomatoes, thinly sliced

1 Tbsp. olive oil

1 ½ Tbsp. apple cider vinegar

1 tsp. dried oregano

½ tsp. dried basil

¼ tsp. sea salt

Mix oil, vinegar, sea salt and oregano. Layer tomatoes in bowl with marinade. Allow to marinate for a few hours, stirring gently on occasion.

Variation: Brussel sprouts, beets, and other vegetables can be marinated in this way (the harder the vegetable, the longer the amount of time to marinate).

Tomato and Onion Salad

3 tomatoes, sliced

1 large sweet onion,
   sliced

¼ cup snipped fresh basil

2 Tbsp. apple cider vinegar

2 Tbsp. olive oil

2 tsp. honey

pinch sea salt

Mix ingredients on right and pour over ingredients on left. Allow to marinate for at least one hour, stirring gently a couple of times before serving.

Broccoli Salad *with Two Dressing Options*

1 bunch broccoli, florets   ¾ cup raisins

¼ red/sweet onion, minced   ½ cup walnuts

Mayonnaise-based Dressing

½ cup mayonnaise ((pg. 100)   2-3 tsp. honey

2 tsp. apple cider vinegar   ¼ tsp. cinnamon

   or lemon juice   pinch sea salt

Mix mayonnaise, vinegar (or lemon), honey, sea salt and cinnamon. Add to chopped broccoli, onion, raisins and nuts. Mix well and allow to chill for at least 2 hours.

Nut/Seed-based Dressing

½ cup almonds or sunflower seeds (presoak at least 8 hours)

2 Tbsp. lemon juice   ¼ - $^1/_3$ cup water

¼ cup dates, pitted   ¼ tsp. cinnamon

3 apricots   ¼ tsp. sea salt

2 Tbsp. olive oil

Process all ingredients in blender until smooth. Combine with chopped broccoli, onion, raisins and nuts.

Cucumber Salad

3 cucumbers, thinly sliced

2 Tbsp. mayonnaise (pg. 100)

1 Tbsp. lemon juice

½ tsp. dill weed

pinch of sea salt

opt: ¼ cup chives
        or diced red onion

Gently mix together all ingredients and allow to marinate at least one hour before serving.

Blended Salad

For most people, the first time they hear of or see a blended salad, they think "Yuck". But those who venture to try one usually enjoy it. A blended salad is simply a green salad added to a blender and processed to the desired consistency. Some of the benefits of a blended salad are less chewing and increased assimilation of nutrients for the consumer.

It's nice to add a tomato and/or avocado to a blended salad for the flavor and creaminess they contribute. A blended salad can also be topped with dressing and garnishes.

Tabouli

1 cup quinoa	¾ tsp. sea salt
½ bunch parsley (1 ½ cup)	¼ tsp. cinnamon
1-2 tomatoes, chopped	¼ tsp. allspice
1 cucumber, diced	juice of 1 lemon
2 green onions, thinly sliced	$^1/_3$ cup olive oil

opt: 2 Tbsp. chopped mint (or ½ tsp. dried mint)

PREP: Rinse quinoa well then cover with water. Drain and rinse 3 times during the first day of soaking. Sprouts should begin forming within the first 24 hours, but you can continue to soak for up to 36-48 hours, if desired.

Finely chop parsley and mix with other ingredients. Add to well-drained quinoa. Allow to chill for an hour before serving.

*Nice served on its own, on a bed of greens
or stuffed in a cored tomato.*

"Create Your Own" Grain Salad

Begin with sprouted quinoa or sweet brown rice.
Add any combination of:

    chopped, grated, diced vegetables
    nuts or seeds   *dried fruit*

and mix with your choice of dressing, mayonnaise or sauce.

Dressings

Oils for Dressings

Extra virgin olive oil (preferably organic) and unrefined oils from nuts and seeds you would consume (sunflower, sesame, flax, etc.) are the best choices for oils in salad dressings. All unrefined oils are rich in essential fatty acids which are healthful to your body. I often refer to them as "good oils". The good fats are sensitive to light, heat and air, however, and should only be used for cold applications (making dressings, drizzling over salads, etc.).

I prefer to use olive oil for dressings that I am going to store and use over a period of time and reserve the use of delicate oils (like flax and good oil blends) for making small batches of dressing that will be used in their entirety at one meal or for adding directly to my salad.

Parsley Garlic Dressing

juice of 1 lemon
2 garlic cloves
½ tsp. sea salt

2 cups chopped parsley
½ cup olive oil

Combine in blender.

Great on grated or shredded cabbage as well as green salads.

Italian Dressing

Juice of 1 lemon

¼ cup apple cider vinegar

¾ cup olive oil

1-2 tsp. honey

½ tsp. garlic powder

½ tsp. onion powder

1 tsp. sea salt

½ tsp. ground mustard

½ tsp. dried oregano

½ tsp. dried basil

¼ tsp. paprika

opt: ½ tsp. kelp

Combine in bottle and shake to mix. This simple dressing is great for marinating vegetables and for use on grain salads.

Garlic Caesar Dressing

juice of 2 lemons

1 Tbsp. prepared mustard

2 Tbsp. apple cider vinegar

opt: ½ tsp. dried basil

15 garlic cloves

½ tsp. sea salt

pinch cayenne

$^1/_3$ cup olive oil

Puree in blender or processor.

Don't be scared off by the number of garlic cloves-
this makes one tasty and zippy dressing!

Creamy Caesar Dressing

¾ cup sunflower seeds

juice of 1 lemon

1 cup water

5 garlic cloves

2 Tbsp. apple cider vinegar

2 tsp. prepared mustard

¼ tsp. kelp powder

¼ tsp. turmeric

1 tsp. sea salt

$^1/_3$ cup olive oil

opt: 1 tsp. honey

PREP: Presoak seeds for at least 6 hours, then drain.

Process all ingredients, except for olive oil, in blender until smooth. Gently blend in olive oil.

Caesar Salad

Grind pumpkin seeds in a coffee grinder or food processor, then toss with prepared Romaine lettuce before topping with the dressing above or **Garlic Caesar Dressing** on page 89.

Sweet and Sour Dressing

$^1/_3$ cup apple cider vinegar   ¾ tsp. paprika

$^1/_3$ cup honey   ¾ tsp. ground mustard

¼ small onion $^1/_3$ cup olive oil

½ tsp. sea salt   opt: 1 tsp. celery seeds

Puree all (except oil and seeds) in blender. Gently blend in oil (and seeds, if including) when done.

Herb Dressing

¼ sweet/red onion   1 tsp. sea salt

1 garlic clove   ½ tsp. ground cumin

2-3 dates, pitted   ½ tsp. dried basil

2 tsp. prepared mustard   ½ tsp. dried oregano

juice of 1 lemon   ½ tsp. kelp powder

½ cup water   opt: pinch of cayenne

        ¼ cup olive oil

Process all but oil in blender until smooth. Gently blend in oil.

Tahini Dressing

$^1/_3$ cup tahini (pg. 100)		1-2 garlic cloves
juice of 1 lemon		½ tsp. sea salt
½ cup water		pinch of cayenne
¾ tsp. ground mustard	**-or-**	¾ tsp. paprika
¼ cup fresh parsley	**-or-**	¼ small onion
½ cup olive oil		opt: 1 fresh tomato

Blend tahini, lemon, water and garlic cloves until smooth. Add rest of ingredients and blend until mixed.

Honey Mustard Dressing

¼ cup prepared mustard	¼ cup tahini (pg. 100)
$^1/_3$ cup honey	¼ cup water
¼ cup apple cider vinegar	½ cup olive oil

Mix ingredients (except for olive oil) in blender. Gently blend in olive oil. Refrigerate.

Ginger Sesame Dressing

1 ½ Tbsp. fresh ginger

1-2 garlic cloves

¼ cup tahini (pg. 100)

juice of 1 lemon (or 3 Tbsp.
    apple cider vinegar)

1 Tbsp. honey

1 Tbsp. prepared mustard

¾ tsp. sea salt

¼ cup water

pinch of cayenne

½ cup olive oil

opt: 2 Tbsp. sesame seeds

Process all but olive oil and sesame seeds in blender until smooth. Gently blend in olive oil and sesame seeds.

Sweet Oriental-Style Dressing

½ cup apricots

3 Tbsp. tahini (pg. 100)

1 Tbsp. fresh ginger

1 tsp. prepared mustard

2 Tbsp. apple cider vinegar

¾ cup water

¾ tsp. sea salt

½ cup olive oil

3 Tbsp. sesame seeds

Combine all ingredients, except oil and sesame seeds, in a blender. Process until smooth. Gently blend in oil and seeds. Add more water if you'd like a thinner consistency.

Tangy Tomato Dressing

1 large tomato	- **or** -	1 cup of cherry tomatoes
8 sun-dried tomato halves		½ tsp. paprika
½ cup tomato soak water		½ tsp. ground mustard
3 Tbsp. apple cider vinegar		¾ tsp. sea salt
$^1/_3$ cup honey		½ cup olive oil
1 tsp. onion powder		opt: 1-2 tsp. celery seed
½ tsp. garlic powder		

PREP: Presoak sun-dried tomatoes for at least 1 hour. Process all ingredients in blender, except for olive oil and celery seed, till smooth. Gently blend in oil (and celery seed).

Cucumber Dill Dressing

2 cucumbers, peeled	1 tsp. onion powder
juice of 1 lemon	½ tsp. ground mustard
¼ cup sunflower seeds	½ cup olive oil
½ tsp. sea salt	1 Tbsp. dill weed

Blend together all ingredients except for oil and dill, until smooth. Gently mix in oil and dill. Refrigerate for several hours before using.

Sunflower Tomato Dressing

¾ cup sunflower seeds

1 tomato

6 sun-dried tomato halves

juice of 1 lemon

1 Tbsp. apple cider vinegar

1 ¼ cup water

1 tsp. sea salt

1 ½ tsp. paprika

1 tsp. garlic powder

2 tsp. onion powder

pinch cayenne

½ cup olive oil

opt: 1 tsp. honey

or 6-8 raisins

PREP: Presoak sunflower seeds for at least 6 hours. Process all ingredients, except for olive oil, in blender until very smooth. Gently blend in olive oil.

Creamy Avocado Dressing

1 avocado

juice of 1 lemon

2 Tbsp. flax oil

3 Tbsp. water

½ tsp. sea salt

½ tsp. dill weed

¼ tsp. dried basil

pinch of curry powder

pinch of cayenne

opt: 1 tomato, 1 cucumber

Blend together in blender or food processor. Use immediately.

Garlic Ranch Dressing

1 ¼ cup sunflower seeds

juice of 2 lemons

1 garlic clove

2 Tbsp. tahini (pg. 100)

1 ½ tsp. sea salt

½ tsp. onion powder

1 ¾ cup water

$^1/_3$ cup olive oil

¾ tsp. dried basil

½ tsp. dried oregano

½ tsp. dried thyme

PREP: Presoak sunflower seeds for at least 6 hours.

Blend ingredients in left column with water in right column. When smooth, gently blend in oil and herbs. This dressing is best if made ahead, so the herbs have time to contribute their flavor.

Creamy Dill Dressing

Make **Garlic Ranch Dressing** (above) and add 1 Tbsp. of dill weed in place of other herbs.

Sauces and Condiments

Sauces and Condiments, cont.

Sunflower Sour Cream

¾ cup sunflower seeds   ½ tsp. sea salt
juice of 1 lemon (¼ cup)   1 tsp. onion powder
½+ cup water   ¼ tsp. garlic powder
1 Tbsp. olive oil

Ideally, presoak sunflower seeds for at least 6 hours (add ½+ cup more water if you haven't). Drain and then puree with the rest of the ingredients in a blender until quite smooth.

Serve topped with fresh chopped chives, if desired.

French Onion Dip

1 ½ tsp. onion powder (addit.)   ½ tsp. poultry seasoning
$^1/_3$ cup dried onion flakes   ¼ tsp. kelp granules

Prepare **Sunflower Sour Cream** (above) and add ingredients above (add fresh minced dill or chives, if desired).

Great as a dip for flax crackers,
Potato Chips *(pg.171) and cut veggies.*

99

Mayonnaise

1 cup almonds
¾ cup water
juice of 1 lemon (¼ cup)
1 tsp. apple cider vinegar
Opt: 1 tsp. honey

¾ tsp. onion powder
¼ tsp. ground mustard
1 ½ - 2 tsp. sea salt
1 cup olive/flax oil

PREP: Presoak almonds for at least 8 hours.

Puree all ingredients in blender, except for oil. When mixture is quite smooth, gently blend in oil (adding more water, if necessary, to reach correct consistency). **Opt:** For lighter mayonnaise, peel almonds before adding to blender.

Tahini

4 cups sesame seeds
1 cup olive oil

½ tsp. sea salt

Begin with frozen sesame seeds (to protect from overheating) and process all in a heavy-duty blender until very smooth. Refrigerate in jars. *(Do not attempt with a standard blender).*

Ketchup/ BBQ Sauce

½ cup dates, pitted

8 sun-dried tomato halves

1 fresh tomato

$^{1}/_{8}$ -¼ sweet/red onion

1 garlic clove

2 Tbsp. olive oil

2 tsp. apple cider vinegar

1 tsp. sea salt

1 tsp. dried basil

2 pinches ground cloves

PREP: Presoak sun-dried tomatoes and dates in ½ cup water for at least 1 hour.

Puree all ingredients (including soak water) in blender until smooth. Keeps for 2-3 days in refrigerator.

Great served with nut loaves and burgers.
Also great added to them just before dehydrating.

Marinara Sauce

12 sun-dried tomato halves   ¼ cup olive oil

4-5 dates, pitted   1 Tbsp. lemon juice

2-3 fresh tomatoes   1 tsp. sea salt

¼ sweet/red onion   ½ tsp. dried oregano

1 garlic clove   1 tsp. dried basil

¼ cup tomato soak water   (or ½ cup fresh basil)

                                      opt: pinch cayenne

PREP: Presoak sun-dried tomatoes and dates in water for at least 1 hour before using. (Reserve soak water).

For smooth sauce: Puree all ingredients together in blender, except herbs. Mix in herbs and allow to sit for at least 1 hour before serving.

For chunky sauce: Coarse chop fresh tomatoes in food processor, then put aside in a bowl. Process rest of ingredients as smooth as possible, then add to bowl with tomatoes. Allow to sit for at least one hour before serving.

For thicker sauce: Leave out ¼ cup soak water.

You can substitute 3 cups of cherry tomatoes or 5-6 Roma tomatoes for the 2-3 fresh tomatoes.

Simple Tomato Sauce

3 tomatoes
1 garlic clove
1 date, pitted

2 Tbsp. olive oil
½ tsp. sea salt
opt: ¼ tsp. dried oregano
¼ tsp. dried basil

Process garlic on its own in processor before adding tomatoes and date. Process, then drain off excess liquid (enjoy this tasty tomato juice!). Add rest of ingredients and process until smooth. *Try substituting some tasty cherry tomatoes!*

Creamy Tomato Sauce

10 sun-dried tomato halves
2 dates, pitted
½ cup tomato soak water
1 garlic clove
½ cup cherry tomatoes
1 tsp. apple cider vinegar

¼ cup sunflower seeds
2 Tbsp. tahini (pg. 100)
juice of 1 lemon
2 Tbsp. olive oil
½ tsp. sea salt
¾ tsp. dried basil

Process all ingredients in blender until smooth. Substitute ½ tomato or 1 Roma tomato for cherry tomatoes.
Serve over veggie pasta and chopped veggies.

Creamy Pasta Sauce

$^1/_3$ cup tahini (pg. 100)   2 Tbsp. olive oil

½ cup nuts   juice of 1 lemon

¾ cup fresh parsley (or basil)   ¼ tsp. sea salt

1 garlic clove   opt: ½ tsp. dried oregano

PREP: Presoak nuts (almonds, walnuts, pine nuts, etc.) for at least 6-8 hours.

Process all until smooth in a food processor or blender, adding parsley (or basil) towards the end of processing. Serve over veggie pasta (see page 140 for options).

Garlic and Oil Sauce

3 garlic cloves   ¼ tsp. sea salt

¼ cup olive oil   opt: pumpkin seeds

Process garlic in food processor until well-minced. Add olive oil and sea salt, and process until well-blended. Drizzle over veggie pasta. Grind pumpkin seeds in a coffee grinder or blender and sprinkle over pasta and sauce.   *Zippy!*

Pesto

4 large garlic cloves   ½ tsp. sea salt

1 ½ cup fresh basil leaves $^1/_3$ cup olive oil

1 Tbsp. lemon juice $^1/_3$ cup nuts (pine nuts,
                                                      walnuts, soaked almonds)

Blend garlic, basil, lemon juice and sea salt in food processor until it forms a paste. Slowly add olive oil. Serve over veggie pasta or grain salad, and sprinkle with chopped nuts.

Extra sauce can be frozen in ice cube trays, and stored in resealable freezer bags in the freezer for up to 3 months.

Winter Pesto *(when fresh basil isn't available)*

2 cups spinach   ½ tsp. sea salt

1 Tbsp. dried basil $^1/_3$ cup olive oil

4 doves garlic $^1/_3$ cup nuts (pine nuts,

1 Tbsp. lemon juice   walnuts, soaked almonds)

Prepare as directed above.

Variation: Replace some spinach with ½ cup of fresh parsley

105

Thai-style Sauce

½ cup almonds

2-3 Tbsp. tahini (pg. 100)

juice of 1 lime

3 garlic cloves

¼ - $^1/_3$ cup dates (to taste)

1-2 Tbsp. fresh ginger

3 Tbsp. olive oil

¼ cup water

½ tsp. sea salt

pinch- $^1/_8$ tsp. cayenne

PREP: Presoak almonds for at least 8 hours.

Puree well in blender. Serve over Thai-style pasta (below).

Add a little water and oil to modify into a dressing.

Thai-style Veggie Pasta

2 zucchini

1 yellow squash

1 carrot

3 green onions

½ red pepper

opt: chopped cilantro

Spiral-slice zucchini, yellow squash and carrot. Thinly slice green onions and red pepper. Toss spiral-sliced veggies with Thai-style sauce, then arrange in an attractive mound on dinner plates, topped with green onions and peppers (and cilantro). **Optional:** Sprinkle with chopped almonds.

Sweet and Sour Sauce

juice of 1 orange

juice of ½ lemon

$^1/_3$ cup dates, pitted

1 Tbsp. fresh ginger

¼ tsp. ground mustard

1 Tbsp. olive oil

½ tsp. sea salt

1 tsp. psyllium powder

opt: 2 dried apricots

or 1 Tbsp. honey

Blend all ingredients until smooth in a blender.

Variation: Add 1 tsp. curry powder for a curry-style sweet and sour sauce.

To make into a dressing   Add another ½ tsp. sea salt, ¼ cup olive oil and ¼- ½ cup water.

Sweet and Sour Vegetables

Combine and marinate any combination of the following in the sauce above:

broccoli- small florets

bok choy/Napa cabbage-
    thin slices

zucchini- thin strips

pea pods

green onions- slice on diagonal

carrots- slice thinly on diagonal

jicama- thin slices

red pepper- thin slices

opt: sliced soaked almonds

Salsa

2 large tomatoes **or** 5 Romas **or** 2 cups cherry tomatoes

6 sun-dried tomato halves   juice of 1 lemon or lime

2 shallots (¼ sweet onion)   2 tsp. apple cider vinegar

¼ red bell pepper   ¾ tsp. sea salt

1 garlic clove   opt: 1-2 tsp. honey

1-3 tsp. minced jalapeno   ½ cup chopped cilantro

PREP: Presoak sun-dried tomatoes for at least 1 hour.
If using an onion, briefly soak chopped onion in water to mellow intensity, if desired.

Chop each vegetable individually in food processor. Add to bowl. Drain juice from chopped vegetables from bowl into blender. Add garlic, jalapeno, lemon/lime juice, vinegar, sea salt, and honey. Process until smooth. Combine with chopped vegetables and add chopped cilantro. Allow to sit for at least one hour to allow flavors to blend.

Option: Substitute a pinch of cayenne for the jalapeno.

*Great served with flax crackers, in burritos
and tacos (pg. 148), and to top other raw entrees.*

108

Tropical Salsa

To **Salsa** recipe (pg. 108), add chopped pineapple and/or mango. Top with plenty of chopped cilantro.

Guacamole

2 avocados

¼ - ½ onion*, minced

1 fresh tomato, diced

juice of ½ lemon

2 Tbsp. olive oil

¼ - ½ tsp. sea salt

pinch cayenne

opt: 1 chopped garlic clove

2 Tbsp. chopped cilantro

Slice avocado in half lengthwise. Gently twist 2 halves apart. Grip pit with knife blade and gently pop out (reserve pit to add to guacamole if storing before serving- this will help preserve the fresh green color). Scoop avocado out of skin. Mash with a fork. Add rest of ingredients and mix together.

*sweet or red onion (unless you like spicy!)

Variation: The juice of 1 lime can be used in place of the lemon juice.

Raisin Chutney

2 cups raisins

juice of 1 lemon

1-2 Tbsp. fresh ginger

¼- ½ tsp. cloves

2 pinches cayenne

2 pinches sea salt

opt: 1-2 tsp. honey,

to taste

Rinse raisins with boiling water, then soak briefly. Drain, then process with rest of ingredients in blender.

Can be refrigerated for up to 2 weeks.

To ½ batch of chutney, add any or all of the following:

1-2 tomatoes- peeled, seeded and finely chopped

1 peeled, cored and finely chopped apple or pear

¼ red/sweet onion, finely chopped

Honey Mustard Sauce

¼ cup tahini (pg. 100)

2-4 Tbsp. honey

1 ½ Tbsp. prepared mustard

½ tsp. ground mustard

¾ tsp. sea salt

opt: 1 Tbsp. water

Whisk ingredients together. Store in refrigerator.

Excellent spread on burgers and used in making nori rolls.

Cranberry Chutney

12 oz. fresh cranberries (1 bag)	½ cup raw honey
2 oranges (1 peeled)	1 tsp. grated ginger
1 apple, cored and peeled	½ tsp. ground cloves
opt: 2 cups pineapple	1 cup chopped walnuts

Seed oranges. Coarsely chop cranberries in food processor, then add to a bowl. Add rest of ingredients to processor (except walnuts) and coarsely chop. Combine with cranberries and walnuts in bowl.

A great holiday side dish and sauce.
Very nice served with nut loaf.

My mother-in-law and I have enjoyed it
straight from the bowl (as a fruit salad!).

Dips and Fillings

Dips and Fillings, cont.

Many dips and fillings have
presoaked nuts and seeds as a base.

Recipes that include **presoaked almonds** will require less planning ahead if you keep a jar of them on hand in the refrigerator. Recipes including **sunflower and pumpkin seeds** suggest a six-hour soaking period for optimal germination (and improved digestion and assimilation), but these can be prepared with seeds that have been soaked for as little as one hour (or with dry seeds when additional water is added). Any recipes that require **a combination of nuts/seeds** that soak for varying amounts of time can be soaked together for the longest recommended time.

Uses for Dips and Fillings

Added to the top or side of salads.

Rolled in lettuce leaves, cabbage or Napa leaves.

Stuffed in celery sticks, tomatoes, avocados, peppers, etc.

Rolled in nori sheets.

Used as a dip with cut veggies, dehydrated veggie chips or crackers.

Stuffers	*Roll-ups*
tomatoes	lettuce leaves
zucchini	spinach leaves
yellow squash	cabbage leaves
avocados	Napa cabbage leaves
sweet onions	collard leaves
bell peppers	chard leaves
celery	untoasted nori

Dippers

celery sticks	radishes
carrot sticks	cherry tomatoes
baby carrots	cucumber slices
zucchini sticks	red pepper strips
sliced turnip	mushrooms
sliced jicama	broccoli/cauliflower
dehydrated veggie chips	flax crackers

Lettuce Roll-ups

Spread the **dip or filling** of your choice onto a lettuce leaf. **Add** grated vegetables, sliced avocado, chopped tomato, sprouts, etc. Simply **roll up and enjoy** or additionally add a drizzle of flax oil (or other good oils), dressing or a sauce.

Nori Rolls

Place untoasted nori sheet on dry cutting board and layer a strip of the following additions within a couple of inches of one edge. Roll nori with fillings into a tight roll. Dampen edge and seal shut. Serve as is or slice into pieces.

Nori roll additions:

avocado	thin cucumber sticks
sliced tomatoes	spinach leaves
grated carrot	sliced green onions
grated zucchini, yellow squash	fresh herbs:
grated Jerusalem artichokes	cilantro, parsley,
thinly sliced red peppers	basil, dill, etc.

Nori roll seasonings/sauces for drizzling and dipping:

lemon juice	honey mustard sauce
sea salt	sweet and sour sauce

Sunflower Filling

2 cups sunflower seeds

2 garlic cloves

2 Tbsp. tahini (pg. 100)

2 Tbsp. olive oil

juice of 1 lemon

2 tsp. ground cumin

1 ½ tsp. paprika

¼ tsp. kelp powder

¾ tsp. sea salt

PREP: Presoak sunflower seeds for at least 6 hours

Process all ingredients in food processor until fairly smooth.

Fresh Veggie Dip

2 zucchini

$^1/_8$ red/sweet onion

4 garlic cloves

¼ cup fresh parsley

juice of 1 lemon

¼ cup tahini (pg. 100)

2 Tbsp. olive oil

1 tsp. ground cumin

½ tsp. sea salt

opt: 1 tsp. dill weed

Process all ingredients in a food processor until smooth.

Optional additions: Blend in spinach leaves (for spinach dip) or presoaked sunflower seeds (for a creamier dip).

Sunflower Seed Dip

½ cup sunflower seeds   1-2 garlic cloves

¼ cup tahini (pg. 100)   ¼ cup water

juice of one lemon   ¼ tsp. sea salt

$^1/_8$ - ¼ cup sweet/red onion   opt: pinch cayenne

PREP: Presoak sunflower seeds for at least 6 hours.

Puree all ingredients in a food processor or blender (add additional water, if needed).

Option: Add ¼ cup chopped parsley and/or 2 Tbsp. olive oil.

Pumpkin Seed Dip

1 cup pumpkin seeds   ¼ tsp. sea salt

1 cup fresh parsley   pinch cayenne

1 garlic clove   juice of 1 lemon

1-2 Tbsp. fresh ginger   2 Tbsp. olive oil

PREP: Presoak pumpkin seeds for at least 6 hours.

Drain seeds, then blend all ingredients in food processor or blender until well-chopped (as coarse/smooth as you'd like).

"Recycled Dip" Dressing

This is the answer to the question of what to do with what's left clinging to the inside of the blender after making a dip.

Add to blender and whip together:

1 Tbsp. apple cider vinegar

¼ cup water

¼ cup olive oil

¼ tsp. sea salt

pinch of basil

pinch of dill weed

¼ tsp. garlic powder

opt: ¼ tsp. kelp

Tahini Parsley Dip

½ cup tahini (pg. 100)

juice of one lemon

¹/₃ cup water

2 garlic cloves

¼ tsp. sea salt

¹/₃ cup chopped parsley

Whisk together ingredients in left column. Pound garlic with sea salt, then add to mixture. Gently mix in chopped parsley. You can also add some olive oil, if desired.

Variation: To make this dip into a **salad dressing**, dilute with some olive oil and water.

Hummus

3 cups presoaked chickpeas

3 garlic cloves

$^1/_3$ cup tahini (pg. 100)

½ cup sunflower seeds

½ cup water

2+ Tbsp. olive oil

juice of 3 lemons

¾ tsp. ground cumin

1 ½ tsp. sea salt

optional additions:

 ½ tomato

 slice of red onion

 1 red pepper

 ½ cup fresh parsley

PREP: Presoak chickpeas in water for 2-3 days (begin with about 2 cups of chickpeas to produce 3 cups of presoaked beans for recipe). Presoak sunflower seeds in water for at least 6 hours.

Puree all ingredients together in a food processor or heavy-duty blender until smooth. Check flavor and add more lemon, salt or tahini, to taste. Add more water, if needed, to allow the ingredients to circulate more smoothly in the blender. If adding optional ingredients, you may want to reduce the overall amount of water in the recipe.

Spinach Dip

¾ cup sunflower seeds

1 tomato

1 avocado

½ cup water

juice of 1 lemon

¼ cup fresh parsley

1 Tbsp. tahini (pg. 100)

2 tsp. onion powder

½ tsp. ground mustard

1 tsp. sea salt

3 Tbsp. olive oil

½ tsp. dill weed

pinch cayenne

1 bunch spinach

opt: 2 Tbsp. dried onion

PREP: Presoak sunflower seeds for at least 6 hours.

Process sunflower seeds with the rest of the ingredients (except for spinach) in a blender. Spinach can be chopped then added at end, or simply added to mixture towards end of processing for a finer blend.

Variation: Add grated carrot, finely chopped pepper, celery, and sweet onion to the dip after processing.

Sprouted Pea Dip

1 cup dry whole peas

4 carrots, shredded

¾ sweet/red onion

2 garlic cloves

½ cup tahini (pg. 100)

2 Tbsp. olive oil

1 ½ tsp. sea salt

1 Tbsp. ground cumin

1 tsp. turmeric

juice of 2 lemons

PREP: Follow soaking/sprouting directions for whole peas.
1 cup dry peas equals about 1 quart sprouted.

Puree all ingredients together in food processor or heavy-duty blender until smooth.

*Any excess of this recipe can be dehydrated into crackers (much like the **Veggie Crackers** on page 180).*

Sunflower Carrot Filling

1 cup sunflower seeds

1 cup carrot pulp*

¼ red/sweet onion

2 garlic cloves

juice of 1 lemon

¼ cup tahini (pg. 100)

¼ cup water

1 Tbsp. olive oil

½ tsp. sea salt

pinch cayenne

opt: ½ cup fresh parsley

PREP: Reserve 1 cup of carrot pulp from juicing. Presoak sunflower seeds for at least 6 hours.

Process all ingredients in food processor until uniformly mixed.

* or grated carrots

Great stuffed in tomatoes and avocados
and rolled in lettuce leaves and nori rolls.

Simple Almond Dip

1 cup almonds

1 tomato

$^1/_8$ - ¼ sweet/red onion

¼ tsp. turmeric

¼ tsp. sea salt

opt: 1 garlic clove

PREP: Presoak almonds for at least 8 hours

Process all ingredients, except for almonds, in blender. Add almonds and process until smooth.

Fine Almond Dip

Add to recipe above:

additional $^1/_8$ sweet/red onion

¼ red pepper

2 celery ribs

addit. ¼ tsp. sea salt

2 Tbsp. lemon juice

1+ tsp. granulated kelp

opt: ½ cup carrot pulp*

Process these additional ingredients with ingredients for the **Simple Almond Dip** (above).

* Reserve carrot pulp from juicing, or grate carrots.

This dip has a bit of a seafood-like flavor.

Southwestern Dip

1 cup almonds

1 cup sunflower seeds

¼ cup tahini (pg. 100)

1 tomato, chopped

4 sun-dried tomato halves

2 garlic cloves

$^1/_3$ red/sweet onion

1 celery rib, chopped

2 Tbsp. olive/flax oil

2 Tbsp. apple cider vinegar

1 Tbsp. ground cumin

1 Tbsp. chili powder

½ tsp. granulated kelp

½ tsp. dried oregano

½ tsp. sea salt

pinch cayenne

opt: ½ red pepper

PREP: Presoak almonds at least 8 hours, sunflower seeds at least 6 hours, and sun-dried tomatoes at least 1 hour.

Process all ingredients in food processor until fairly smooth.

Dips and Fillings are versatile and can be served:

- with salad
- as a dip
- rolled in leaves of romaine lettuce or Napa cabbage
- stuffed in celery sticks, bell pepper halves, tomato halves and avocado halves

Curried Filling

½ cup walnuts

½ cup sunflower seeds

½ cup pumpkin seeds

2 garlic cloves

¼ - ½ red/sweet onion

¼ red pepper

2 celery ribs

1 Tbsp. lemon juice

½ - 1 tsp. curry powder

2 tsp. ground cumin

2 tsp. turmeric

1 tsp. dried thyme

½ tsp. sea salt

1 Tbsp. olive oil

opt: 1 Tbsp. tahini

opt: ¼ cup fresh parsley

PREP: Presoak walnuts and seeds for at least 6 hours.

Rinse and drain soaked nuts and seeds. Process garlic on its own in processor. Add rest of vegetables and seasonings and process until smooth. Add seeds and nuts and process again until smooth.

Excellent stuffed in tomatoes and avocados and topped with **Salsa** *(pg. 108) or* **Simple Tomato Sauce** *(pg. 103).*

Walnut/Pecan Filling

$^1/_3$ cup sunflower seeds

1 cup walnuts/pecans

1 cup carrot pulp*

$^1/_8$ sweet onion

1 celery rib

½ cup fresh parsley

1 tsp. lemon juice

opt: 2 sun-dried tomato halves

2 Tbsp. olive oil

½ tsp. poultry seasoning

½ tsp. dried basil

½ tsp. garlic powder

½ tsp. granulated kelp

¾ tsp. sea salt

1-3 Tbsp. of water

(as needed)

PREP: Presoak walnuts/pecans for at least 4-6 hours and sunflower seeds for at least 6 hours.

When juicing carrots or a combination of carrots and celery, reserve aside 1 cup of the pulp left from juicing.

Process all ingredients in food processor until well-chopped (not completely smooth), adding only as much water as necessary to allow it to blend together.

* or grated carrots

*This filling is great stuffed in avocado halves and topped with **Salsa** (pg. 108) and chopped cilantro. Looks and tastes beautiful!*

Sunflower Cheese

²/₃ cup sunflower seeds   1 Tbsp. olive oil

½ cup almonds   ¾ tsp. turmeric

½ cup water   ½ tsp. paprika

juice of 1 lemon   ¾ tsp. sea salt

3 Tbsp. tahini (pg. 100)   pinch cayenne

Opt: 3 presoaked sun-dried tomato halves

PREP: Presoak almonds for at least 8 hours, sunflower seeds for at least 6 hours and tomatoes for at least 1 hour.

Puree all ingredients together until smooth.

Serve as a dip with a Mexican-style entrée or flax crackers. This recipe can also be dehydrated into cheese crackers (see directions on page 181).

Cultured Almond Cheese

Presoak almonds.   Puree with water.   Add fresh garlic or garlic powder, onion powder and herbs (dill is great) to make a garlic herb spread.   Allow to ferment in a shallow dish at the bottom of the dehydrator at 100 degrees for 6+ hours.

Use as a dip or spread.

Soups

Soups

Raw soups are a creative adventure. Raw soups are simply a combination of vegetables and seasonings, pureed together. Try the ones described here, but also be sure to try your hand at developing your own soup recipes. You'll have some flops, but you'll also stumble into some combinations that are just great.

"Create Your Own" Soup

Puree a variety of vegetables together in your blender- (tomatoes are usually a nice addition- they add juiciness and flavor). To make a creamy vegetable soup, add any of the following:

> *avocado*
>
> *soaked sunflower seeds*
>
> *soaked almonds*

Serve as is, or pour over a bowl of grated or chopped vegetables. Garnish and serve.

Fresh Tomato Soup

2-3 tomatoes, seeded	2 Tbsp. olive oil
thin slice red/sweet onion	½ tsp. sea salt
1 small garlic clove	1 cucumber
12 sun-dried tomato halves	1 zucchini
$^2/_3$ cup water	1 red pepper
1 Tbsp. apple cider vinegar	1 tomato, seeded
1 tsp. lemon juice	opt: 1 tsp. honey

Puree ingredients in left column with olive oil and sea salt in right column. Dice remaining vegetables and mix into tomato puree. Serve as is or topped with snipped cilantro or parsley. **Optional:** Add some fresh basil and/or oregano.

Soup Accompaniments

*Consider serving some dehydrated **crackers or chips**
along with a soup entrée.*

*Dehydrated **seasoned seeds** are nice sprinkled
on top of a soup before serving.*

Herbed Zucchini Soup

4 zucchini	12 sun-dried tomato halves
2-3 tomatoes	2 Tbsp. lemon juice
2 celery rib	2 Tbsp. olive oil
1 carrot	1 cup water
¼ - ½ red/sweet onion	1 tsp. dried basil
2 garlic cloves	1 tsp. dried oregano
½ cup fresh parsley	1 ½ tsp. paprika
or 1 cup spinach	1 tsp. sea salt

Chop vegetables into small chunks. Add to a heavy-duty blender with all ingredients except for basil and oregano. Blend until smooth. Mix in basil and oregano. Chill for at least 1 hour before serving, to allow time for the herbs to contribute their flavor.

Carrot Soup

4-6 carrots

2 celery ribs

$^1/_8$ red/sweet onion

1 garlic clove

¼ cup fresh parsley

   or 1 cup spinach

1 apple, peeled

2 dates, pitted

2 cups water

2 tsp. lemon juice

1 ½ tsp. ground cumin

½ tsp. sea salt

opt: 1 tsp. dill weed

Roughly chop carrots, celery and onion. Process with rest of ingredients in blender until smooth. Serve immediately in bowls garnished with spiral-cut carrot or sprigs of parsley.

Variation: Add 1/3 cup presoaked sunflower seeds for a creamy version.

Sweet Potato Apple Soup

2 small/ 1 large sweet potato
1 sweet apple, peeled and cored
1 tart apple (Granny Smith)
½ tsp. pumpkin pie spice

5 dates, pitted
¾ - 1 cup water
½ tsp. cinnamon
¼ tsp. sea salt

Peel and cut sweet potato into chunks. Process all but sweet potato in blender until well-blended. Drop in sweet potato piece by piece and continue processing until smooth. Add more water if soup is too thick.

Warm Your Soup

Raw soups don't need to be served cold (straight from the refrigerator). Be careful to not warm soups above 105 degrees, however, as the enzymes begin to die soon above that temperature.

Options for warming soups

1. Continue to process soup in blender until soup warms.
2. Place soup in a covered serving bowl in bottom of dehydrator and warm at 100 degrees for 4-6 hours.
3. Place soup in a bowl that can nest within another bowl that contains hot water (punch bowls work well for this).

Butternut Soup

1 butternut squash (about 4 cups, peeled and cubed)

juice of 2 oranges   ¾ cup dates, pitted

$^1/_8$-¼ sweet/red onion   1 tsp. cinnamon

6 sun-dried tomato halves   1 tsp. sea salt

2-3 Tbsp. tahini (pg. 100)

Process all but squash in a heavy-duty blender until well-blended. Add cubed squash, piece by piece, and continue processing until very smooth. Add as much water as you would like to reach desired consistency.

Curried Butternut Soup

Prepare as directed above and add the following ingredients:

    2 cloves of garlic

    1 tsp. fresh ginger

    1 tsp. ground cumin

    about 1 tsp. curry powder (to taste)

Chili

2 tomatoes	1 tsp. sea salt
¼ sweet/ red onion	2 celery ribs, finely diced
4 garlic cloves	2 zucchini, finely diced
20 sun-dried tomato halves	2 ears of corn, cut kernels
½ cup raisins	½ red pepper, finely diced
2 Tbsp. chili powder	1 cup chopped walnuts
2 tsp. ground cumin	opt: 1 grated carrot
1 tsp. dried oregano	opt: 1 chopped tomato
$^{1}/_{3}$ cup olive oil	

PREP: Presoak walnuts for at least 4 hours. Presoak sun-dried tomatoes for at least 1 hour.

Blend ingredients in left column plus sea salt in right column until smooth. Add prepared vegetables and nuts to a large bowl then mix in sauce. Allow to sit for at least 6 hours (overnight works well) to allow for the spices to fully contribute their flavor. If desired, place in a dehydrator at 100 degrees for several hours in advance of serving to warm to a pleasing temperature.

For a chunkier chili: Process ingredients in left column in a food processor instead of a blender.

Entrées

Entrées, cont.

Nutmeats

Entrée options in other sections of this recipe book:

Salads- marinated vegetables, tabouli, grain salads, etc.

Sauces- Thai-style pasta, sweet and sour veggies, etc.

Dips/Fillings- stuffed veggies, lettuce and nori rolls, etc.

Snacks/Dehydrated Foods- cereals and porridges

Desserts/Treats- ice cream, pies, cookies, etc.

Entrée Options

When it comes to eating an all-raw meal, many people are confused as to what qualifies as an entrée. As discussed in under **Eating Tips** (pg. 37-38), the more you can simplify your meal prep and recipe selection, the easier and more successful you will find raw eating.

We usually begin our **morning** with fresh vegetable **juices** or a **fruit smoothie** (and sometimes fruit for a snack).

Lunch is often a **fruit-based meal** (whole fruit, fruit salad, fruit smoothie/fruit soup) or a **salad-based meal**.

Dinner begins with a large green salad with a wide variety of toppings (there isn't usually a whole lot of belly-room left after that!). The salad can be followed by or coupled with an "entrée". This can be as simple as a **dip or filling** accompanying the salad, or stuffed or rolled into another veggie. Add some dehydrated crackers and this is a very satisfying meal.

Other fairly simple entrées can include:

Burritos, tacos, or **nachos**

Pizza

Pasta with sauce

Nut loaves and **burgers** are a welcome change on occasion
They're not recommended as a regular part of the diet
because of the preparation time involved and the
large amount of rich nuts and seeds

Grain-based salads and **cereals** are also filling meal
options.

Soup, coupled with some dehydrated crackers, is a quick
meal.

Consider having a **dessert night** on occasion
For a special occasion or as a break from the routine,
serve soft-serve ice cream or a fruit smoothie with a
raw pie or cookies.

Veggie Pasta

Use a spiral-slicer to make spaghetti from:

*Zucchini (peeled or with peel)- **most versatile pasta***

Yellow squash (summer, crookneck)

Sweet potato (soak at least 1 hour in water)

Red potato (soak at least 1 hour in water with lemon)

Butternut squash	*Carrot*
Rutabaga or turnip	*Jicama*
Daikon radish	*Beet (as a garnish)*

Add some accent veggies:

Red, yellow or orange bell pepper- into strips or rings

Green onions- into rings

Sweet/red onion- into rings (briefly soak in water or use
   ***Mellowing Marinade** (pg. 78) to mellow the intensity).*

Serve veggie pasta with a dressing, Marinara Sauce, Pesto, Salsa, or another sauce of your choice.

If you don't have a spiral-slicer, you can make veggie pasta by shaving vegetables into thin strips with a vegetable peeler (fettuccini-style) or by grating into shreds. You'll find that the shape of the "noodle" affects the experience of the "pasta".

Pasta Options

Zucchini Pasta served with any of the following:

Marinara Sauce

Simple Tomato Sauce

Creamy Tomato Sauce

Pesto Sauce

Winter Pesto

Creamy Pasta Sauce

Thai-style Sauce

Sweet and Sour Sauce

Salsa

Spiral-sliced zucchini makes an incredible pasta. My husband was pretty skeptical, but willing enough to give it a try. He was pleasantly surprised by how similar the zucchini noodles were to "al dente" angel hair pasta.

Thai-Style Pasta and Sauce   pg. 106

Remember, raw entrees don't need to be served cold.
Allow veggie pasta and sauce to at least warm to
room temperature, or place covered in a
100 degree dehydrator to warm further.

Lasagna

4 zucchini	¼ - ½ sweet/red onion
1 red pepper	2 tomatoes

Slice vegetables as thin as possible on a mandoline slicer. Mix vegetables in marinade (below) until well-coated. Allow to marinate for at least 4 hours, preferably overnight. Drain off liquid when ready to assemble lasagna.

Marinade: Combine the following in a food processor or crush the garlic and whisk with other ingredients in a bowl.

3 garlic cloves	1 tsp. kelp powder
1 Tbsp. lemon juice	1 Tbsp. dried basil
$^1/_3$ cup olive oil	1 tsp. dried oregano
1 tsp. sea salt	½ tsp. dried thyme

Assembling lasagna: Layer marinated vegetables, **Sunflower Ricotta** (pg. 143) and **Marinara Sauce** (pg. 102) in a 9 x 12 pan. Repeat layering once more. (Alternatively, you can add a layer of chopped spinach). Top with **Marinara Sauce** and **Sunflower Parmesan** (pg. 143) or ground pumpkin seeds. Leave at room temperature (or put in dehydrator at 100 degrees) for 2+ hours before serving.

Sunflower Ricotta

2 cups sunflower seeds	1 ½ tsp. onion powder
juice of 1 lemon	¼ tsp. garlic powder
1 Tbsp. tahini (pg. 100)	1 tsp. sea salt
2 Tbsp. olive oil	¾ - 1 cup water

PREP: Presoak sunflower seeds at least 6 hours.

Drain sunflower seeds. Add rest of ingredients and process until smooth. You want to use as little water as possible so the "cheese" stays thick for use.

Reserve some for use in making
Sunflower Parmesan *(below), if desired.*

Sunflower Parmesan

Spread about ¼ cup of **Sunflower Ricotta** (above) very thinly on a piece of parchment paper on a dehydrating sheet. Dehydrate at 100 degrees until thoroughly dry. Remove from sheet and crumble or process in food processor.

Pizza

1 batch of **Pizza Crusts** (pg. 182) or **thick flax crackers**

½ batch **Marinara Sauce** (pg. 102)

Optional cheese toppings:

> **Sunflower Ricotta** (pg. 143)
>
> **Ground pumpkin seeds**

Pizza Assembly:

Top pizza crust with **Marinara Sauce**, then any combination of the following:

> thinly sliced tomatoes
>
> thinly sliced onions (as is or marinate ahead of time)
>
> sliced red, yellow or orange peppers
>
> grated zucchini
>
> grated summer squash

Serve as is, or place in dehydrator for 8-10 hours for a more traditional look, temperature and taste.

When ready to serve, sprinkle with ground pumpkin seeds (like parmesan) or dot with **Sunflower Ricotta** *(pg. 143).*

Vegetable Kabobs

zucchini   sweet onion   mushrooms
summer squash   red bell peppers   cherry tomatoes

Cut veggies into chunks (except for cherry tomatoes) and marinate (in dressing or **Mellowing Marinade**, pg. 78) for at least 6 hours. Poke veggies onto bamboo skewers and put in dehydrator at 100 degrees for at least 6-8 hours.

Broccoli/Cauliflower with Cheese Sauce

1 head broccoli or cauliflower (or a combination of the two)
*1 batch of **Sunflower Dip** or **Sunflower Cheese***
opt: finely diced red pepper

Chop broccoli/cauliflower as large or fine as you would like. Top with **Sunflower Seed Dip** (pg. 117) or **Sunflower Cheese** (pg. 127), then sprinkle with red pepper or paprika. You can dehydrate this dish for a couple of hours before serving if you'd prefer it warm.

*For a less "raw" broccoli or cauliflower flavor, marinate veggies overnight in **Mellowing Marinade** (pg. 78) before draining off excess liquid and adding topping.*

Mashed Potatoes with Sour Cream

1 small head or ½ large head of cauliflower (about 3-5 cups)

¾ cup sunflower seeds   1 tsp. onion powder

¼ cup pecans   ¼ tsp. poultry seasoning

$^1/_3$ cup water   ¼ tsp. dried thyme

3 Tbsp. olive oil   ½ tsp. sea salt

3 Tbsp. lemon juice   opt: chopped chives

PREP: Presoak sunflower seeds and pecans for at least 6 hours.

Process all but cauliflower in a blender until smooth. Add chunks of cauliflower and process again until all is smooth.

This is obviously not prepared with potatoes but cauliflower,
yet the effect is quite similar to mashed potatoes.
Serve as is or with chopped chives.

Curried Cauliflower

1 head cauliflower

½ red pepper

$^1/_3$ cup sunflower seeds

2 Tbsp. tahini (pg. 100)

juice of 1 lemon

¼ red/sweet onion

1 garlic clove

1 Tbsp. olive oil

½ tsp. curry powder

1 tsp. ground cumin

½ tsp. turmeric

½ tsp. sea salt

2 Tbsp. water

PREP: Presoak sunflower seeds in water for at least 6 hours.

Pulse chop cauliflower in food processor until finely chopped. Place in a shallow casserole dish. Finely dice red pepper and mix with cauliflower for colorful presentation or add whole to sauce mixture for simpler preparation. Add rest of ingredients to a blender and puree until very smooth. Stir into cauliflower, then place in dehydrator for at least 2 hours before serving (stirring occasionally) to warm dish.

Tacos and Burritos

Taco- *fold lettuce leaf and fill with additions*

Burrito- *roll additions inside leaf*

Tostada- *layer additions on whole romaine leaves*

Suggested Additions:

Salsa

Guacamole

Sunflower Sour Cream

Sunflower Dip

Pumpkin Seed Dip

Sunflower Carrot Filling

Southwestern Dip

Sunflower Filling

Pecan/Walnut Filling

Sprouted Pea Dip

Simple/Fine Almond Dip

Chopped avocado

Chopped tomatoes

Chopped red peppers

Chopped celery

Grated carrot

Grated zucchini

Grated summer squash

Chopped cilantro

Crummles

Sunflower Cheese

Hummus

Nachos

Large carrots

Jicama

Flax crackers

Turnip/rutabaga

Jerusalem artichokes

Dehydrated crackers

Slice vegetables on mandoline slicer into chip-thickness. Arrange on a plate. Either serve with bowls containing the following options **or** top directly with your choice of:

Salsa

Sunflower Sour Cream

Sunflower Ricotta

Crummles

Sunflower Cheese

Guacamole

Chopped cilantro

Chopped tomatoes

Chopped lettuce

Chopped avocado

Nutmeat Recipes

The flavor depth and richness of nuts and seeds lend more of the taste and texture we expect from burgers and meat loaves. Do not expect any of these to actually trick you into believing they are a fast-food burger, however. But they're certainly tasty and enjoyable in their own right. Because they include such a large amount of nuts and seeds (rich in fats and high in protein) they should be considered "delicacies" in our diet, not staples.

Enjoy nutmeats as a change from the routine, especially for special occasions and at the holidays.

Nutmeats Can Be

- Shaped into burgers or loaves and dehydrated to warm them
- Used as a dip
- Used as a filling/stuffing for vegetables
- Served on a salad bed

Note: To simplify the soaking of combinations of nuts and seeds, soak them together for the longest recommended time. Separate soak times are listed in case you have presoaked nuts already on hand.

Sunflower "Tuna" Salad

½ cup sunflower seeds	1 Tbsp. olive oil
½ cup almonds	$^1/_8$ tsp. garlic powder
1 carrot	¾ tsp. kelp powder
2 celery ribs	½ tsp. sea salt
$^1/_8$ sweet/red onion	opt: ½ tomato
¼ cup fresh parsley	½ red pepper
1 Tbsp. lemon juice	1 chopped green onion

PREP: Presoak almonds for at least 8 hours and sunflower seeds for 6 hours.

Grate carrot and celery into food processor. Add rest of ingredients and process until desired consistency (from coarsely chopped to finely ground). Allow to rest for at least one hour for flavors to blend.

Also great with 2-3 Tbsp. of mayonnaise (pg. 100) added.

Attractively arrange a "Tuna Salad Plate"
Serve a mound of **Sunflower "Tuna" Salad** *on a bed of lettuce, accompanied on dinner plate by ½ avocado and ½ tomato (chopped or whole). Additional vegetable garnishes could be added, as well as a dollop of mayonnaise and sprig of parsley or sprinkle of paprika on top of the tuna salad.*

Nut Loaf

1 cup almonds	2 tsp. dried basil
¾ cup sunflower seeds	1 tsp. dried oregano
¾ cup pumpkin seeds	1 tsp. dried thyme
¾ cup pecans or hazelnuts	½ tsp. poultry seasoning
juice of 1 lemon	½ tsp. garlic powder
$^1/_3$ cup olive oil	1 tsp. kelp powder
up to ¼ cup water	¼ - ½ red/sweet onion
1 tsp. sea salt	2 celery ribs
1 Tbsp. ground sage	opt: ½ red pepper

PREP: Presoak nuts and seeds in water for at least 8 hours.

Cut red onion, celery and pepper into chunks, then coarse chop in a food processor. Put in a large bowl. Puree nuts and seeds with liquids in food processor until fairly smooth. Add seasonings and continue to process until well mixed. Pour into bowl and mix well with chopped vegetables.

Form into 5-6 loaves (about 1- 1 ½ inches thick) on parchment paper on dehydrating trays. Place in dehydrator at 100 degrees for at least 2-4 hours to warm.

Nut Loaf, continued

Spread the tops of the loaves with **Ketchup** or **BBQ Sauce**
(pg. 101) before dehydrating for a nice accent flavor
and the look of an authentic "meat loaf".

*Loaves and burgers can be made
from this **recipe without the use of a dehydrator**.
Simply serve at room temperature.*

*These loaves are a nice option as a holiday entrée, especially
when accompanied by **Cranberry Chutney** (pg. 111).*

*This nut loaf is also great used to
stuff tomatoes, red peppers or avocados.
Be sure to top each with **Ketchup/BBQ Sauce**
and warm in dehydrator for at least 4-6 hours.*

A very tasty dish with a beautiful presentation.

Herbed Loaf

1 cup walnuts

½ cup almonds

½ cup sunflower seeds

1 garlic clove

¼ - ½ red/sweet onion

4 celery ribs (with leaves)

1 Tbsp. lemon juice

1 ½ tsp. ground sage

1 tsp. dried thyme

1$^+$ tsp. poultry seasoning

½ tsp. kelp powder

1 tsp. sea salt

opt: 1 Tbsp. olive oil

PREP: Presoak almonds at least 8 hours. Presoak walnuts and sunflower seeds at least 6 hours.

Process garlic clove on its own in processor. Add chopped onion and sliced celery with rest of seasonings and blend until finely chopped. Add walnuts, almonds and sunflower seeds and process until well-mixed.

This is best dehydrated into loaves *(a very adventurous person might try shaping it into little turkeys!)* for 4-6 hours at 100 degrees. Serve garnished with some parsley and possibly with some **Cranberry Chutney** (pg. 111).

The seasonings in this loaf are reminiscent of roast turkey and dressing!

154

Vegetable Loaf

1 large sweet potato	1 cup almonds
1-2 medium red potatoes	½ cup pecans
1 medium turnip	½ cup walnuts
¼-½ red/sweet onion	1 Tbsp. poultry seasoning
1 carrot	1 tsp. ground sage
4 celery ribs, sliced	1 tsp. dried basil
1 Tbsp. lemon juice	1 tsp. dried thyme
3 Tbsp. olive oil	1 tsp. granulated kelp
1 ½ tsp. sea salt	2 tsp. onion powder

PREP: Presoak almonds for at least 8 hours and pecans and walnuts for at least 6 hours. Drain before using.

Peel potatoes, sweet potato and turnip. Process vegetables and nuts through juicer with the blank attachment installed. Mix rest of ingredients and seasonings into this mixture. Form into loaves on parchment paper on dehydrating trays and dehydrate 4-6 hours at 100 degrees. (**Option:** add ¼-½ of a beet to the vegetable mixture. This lends some sweetness and also a striking color).

Optional: Top with **Ketchup/BBQ Sauce** (pg. 101) before dehydrating and serve with additional Ketchup/BBQ Sauce.

This loaf is not as rich as those made predominantly from nuts but the fact that it includes a higher ratio of vegetables is nutritionally in its favor.

Nut Burgers

1 cup walnuts	2 Tbsp. olive oil
1 cup sunflower seeds	1 tsp. chili powder
1 cup carrot pulp*	2 tsp. onion powder
¼ red/sweet onion	½ tsp. garlic powder
¼ cup fresh parsley	1 tsp. ground cumin
4 sun-dried tomato halves	½ tsp. dried basil
½ cup tomato soak water	½ tsp. poultry seasoning
2 Tbsp. tahini (pg. 100)	1 tsp. sea salt

PREP: Reserve 1 cup of carrot pulp from juicing. Presoak walnuts for at least 4 hours, sunflower seeds for 6 hours, sun-dried tomatoes 1 hour. Reserve soak water for recipe.

Process all ingredients in food processor until uniformly mixed, but not pureed. The mixture should hold together, but not be the consistency of a dip. Shape with your hands into half-inch thick patties and place on parchment paper on dehydrating trays and dehydrate at 100 degrees for at least 4 hours (more for a dryer burger). Flip burgers and remove parchment paper about halfway through dehydrating time. Refrigerate or freeze extra burgers and warm in dehydrator (for at least 2 hours) when ready to serve.

* or grated carrots

Buckwheat Burgers

1 ½ cups buckwheat groats (about 2 cups soaked)

1 cup sunflower seeds   1 tsp. dried oregano

2 carrots   ½ tsp. sage

2 celery ribs   ½ tsp. kelp powder

1 small slice red onion   1 tsp. ground cumin

1 Tbsp. lemon juice   1 tsp. sea salt

¼ tsp. garlic powder

PREP: Soak buckwheat groats for at least 8 hours (rinse and drain before using). Presoak sunflower seeds for at least 1 hour.

Blend all ingredients together in food processor until smooth. Form into ½ inch thick burgers on parchment paper on dehydrating trays and dehydrate at 100 degrees for at least 4 hours (more for a dryer burger). Refrigerate or freeze extra burgers and reheat (at least 2 hours) in dehydrator when ready to serve. *(Note: These burgers have a sharper flavor).*

Burgers are great served with
sliced tomatoes, lettuce, onions, avocado,
ketchup/BBQ sauce, mayonnaise,
honey mustard sauce, salsa and guacamole.

Snacks and Dehydrated Foods

Snacks and Dehydrated Foods

Snacks and Dehydrated Foods

Raw Snacks

Fresh Raw Snacks

Fresh fruit

Fresh fruit juice

Dried fruit

Fruit smoothie

Soft-serve ice cream

Banana-sicles

Nuts/seeds

Nut-stuffed dates

Trail mix

Fresh vegetable juice

Cut veggies and dip

Salad and dressing

Fruit and Nut Cereal

Buckwheat Porridge

Raw Pies

Fruit-and-Nut Truffles

Raw Sweets and Treats

Raw Snacks, *continued*

Dehydrated Raw Snacks

Fruit Leather

Fruit Chips

Vegetable Chips

Flax Crackers

Dehydrated Crackers

Seasoned Seeds

Dehydrated Nuts

Dehydrated Cookies

Buckwheat Crunchies

Granola

Why Dehydrate?

Though dehydration may seem an unfamiliar process, it is actually on of the oldest forms of natural food preservation. Originally, foods were sun-dried but now that we have the convenience of dehydrating machines we can speed the process and don't run the risk of having our foods sampled by critters as they dry in the sun.

Many who consume an entirely raw or predominantly raw diet often miss the "crunch" or "chewiness" of many cooked foods. Using a dehydrator allows you to create crunchy and chewy raw foods.

Dehydration Tips

Dehydrate at **100 degrees** to preserve enzymes (you can safely dehydrate between 90 and 105 degrees, but I like to consistently dehydrate at 100 degrees just because it's easy to remember).

I'm not sure it's possible to over-dehydrate, so I tend to leave things in longer than they might need. Consequently, I'm not very careful about watching for specific **dehydrating times**, so the suggested times are just estimates. Always check for desired consistency/texture/crispness and make a note by the recipe indicating what time worked well for you. Also the amount of items you are dehydrating, whether they begin dehydration on parchment paper and the original moistness will all be factors in dehydrating times.

When **transferring a dehydrating recipe** that began on a sheet of parchment paper to the plain dehydrating tray, simply place a new tray face down on the partly-dehydrated recipe, then flip both trays. Remove original tray and parchment paper. Return new tray to dehydrator.

Transfer your dehydrated snacks to glass containers or resealable **plastic bags** and **store in the refrigerator** until ready to use. It's important to keep moisture out for the longest shelf-life. I tend to take things directly out of the dehydrator, put them in the container, immediately seal it and put it in the refrigerator. Crackers, fruit leathers, etc. will keep a month or more this way. Many dehydrated foods that have all the moisture extracted can be stored in containers in a cool, dark, dry place, but I just prefer to have them within sight and with added protection in the refrigerator. Also, any dehydrated foods including nuts and seeds should be refrigerated to further protect the good oils.

Some basic vegetables can be dehydrated for use in soups and in seasoning dishes:

> *Onion (rings or diced)*
> *Celery (sliced or diced)*
> *Carrots (sliced, diced or grated)*
> *Bell peppers (diced)*
> *Tomatoes (slice)*
> *Parsley (whole, then crumble into flakes)*

*Dehydrating is a great way to **use fruits and vegetables** of which you have an excess or which are in danger of "going by". You can easily slice or puree them and then dehydrate for later use.*

*Dehydrating can be **great fun**. All kinds of creative experimentation can take place in the dehydrator. Any time you have excess of a prepared raw food (dips, fillings, salsa, etc.) you can spread as is on parchment paper or mix with some presoaked flax seeds before spreading onto paper. Chances are good that at the end of dehydration you'll have a tasty cracker or a topping you can crumble and add to salads or other dishes.*

Fruit Leathers

To make fruit leathers, all you basically do is prepare applesauce or a fruit smoothie, spread about ¼ inch thick on a piece of parchment paper on a dehydrating tray, then dehydrate until it releases from the paper (about 8-12 hours).

Adding 1-2 tsp. of lemon juice *helps preserve color and can add a pleasant tang to the final product.*

Apple Fruit Leather

Blend apples until smooth. (Don't bother peeling if organic).

Optional: Add some cinnamon to mixture.

Apple/Pear Fruit Leather

Blend apples and pears in blender (ratio is up to you).

Optional: Add some cinnamon to mixture.

Apple/Strawberry Fruit Leather

Blend apples and strawberries in blender.

Other Apple-Based Fruit Leather Variations:

Add:

dates	*peaches*	*cherries*
blueberries	*apricots*	*grapes*
cranberries	*pineapple*	*plums*

Banana Fruit Leather

Blend very ripe bananas and add a dash of lemon juice. Follow the rest of the directions for fruit leathers on pg. 166.

For variations add:

	cinnamon
apple	*berries*
pineapple	*walnuts*

Banana Nut Bars

5 bananas	*$^1/_3$ cup raisins*
1 tsp. lemon juice	*pinch of sea salt*
½ cup dates, pitted	*1 cup chopped walnuts*

PREP: Presoak raisins and dates. Drain before using.

Process bananas, lemon juice, dates, raisins and sea salt in a blender until smooth. Hand mix in chopped walnuts. Spread thickly (½ inch or more) onto parchment paper on dehydrating sheets. Dehydrate for at least 24-48 hours, until dry enough to tear or cut into bars.

Fruit Chips

Almost any fruit can be sliced and dried into chips. *I've even made watermelon chips!* Just place on trays and dehydrate.

In addition to those included here, try:

> *pear, peach, plum, kiwi, pineapple, mango, etc.*

Banana Chips

Slice bananas a little thicker than ¼ inch. Place individual slices on dehydrating tray. Dehydrate at least 12 hours (can flip halfway through drying time). Dry until chewy or crisp.

Apple Chips

Slice apples about ¼ inch thick. Place individual slices on dehydrating tray. Dehydrate at least 12 hours (can flip halfway through drying time).

Option: Sprinkle with cinnamon before dehydrating.

Caramel Apples

Fresh apples- sliced
Banana chips (dehydrated bananas)

Eat apple slices with dehydrated bananas. The bananas contribute not only a caramel-like flavor, but also the "stick to your teeth" effect we're all familiar with in caramel apples!

This may look too simple, but give it a try.
You'll be surprised how good it is!

Glazed Bananas

3-4 bananas   *1 Tbsp. olive oil*
1-2 Tbsp. honey   *¼ - ½ tsp. cinnamon*

Slice bananas and layer in shallow bowl or on plate. Combine rest of ingredients and drizzle with bananas with glaze. Put on bottom of dehydrator (at 100 degrees) for one hour, stirring once or twice, until nicely softened and warmed.

Serve sprinkled with chopped nuts or
drizzled with **Carob Sauce** *(pg. 217).*

Veggie Chips

Sweet Potato Chips

Peel sweet potatoes (unless the skins are in very good condition). Slice with mandoline slicer (or by hand) a little less than a ¼ inch thick (cut on a diagonal to get longer chips). Cover with water and allow to soak for at least 2 hours (to eliminate some of the starch). Place on dehydrating tray and sprinkle with cinnamon or other seasonings. Dehydrate at least 12 hours (longer to be crisper).

Zucchini/Cucumber/Eggplant Chips

Because these contain so much water, you'll need to slice them thicker than your mandoline slicer may allow- at least ¼ inch thick. Place on dehydrating tray and sprinkle with chili powder, garlic powder and/or onion powder.

The eggplant chips are especially nice when marinated with **Mellowing Marinade** (pg. 78) before dehydration. See directions for **Marinated Eggplant Chips** on page 81.

Potato Chips

3 pounds red potatoes

$^1/_3$ cup olive oil

juice of 2 lemons

2 tsp. sea salt

1 tsp. paprika

1 tsp. ground cumin

1 tsp. onion powder

¼ tsp. garlic powder

Wash red potatoes and cut out any "bad" spots. Slice with mandoline slicer (or by hand) about $^1/_8$ inch thick. Cover with water and the juice of 1 lemon. Allow to soak for at least 3 hours (to eliminate some of the starch). Mix rest of ingredients (oil, juice of other lemon and seasonings) in a large bowl, then briefly toss the potato slices in the bowl. Place in a single layer on dehydrating trays and dehydrate at 100 degrees for 24-36 hours (check for crispness).

Great served with **French Onion Dip** *(pg. 99).*

Dehydrated Crackers

Can be enjoyed in a variety of ways

- On their own, as a snack
- To scoop up salsa, guacamole and dips
- As pizza crusts (make a little thicker in this case)
- To make "sandwiches"- spread with filling or sauce and add lettuce, avocado, sliced tomato and any other veggies

Flax seeds are an instrumental ingredient when making great crackers. When flax seeds soak they form a gelatinous substance that works to bind the ingredients together. Cracker "batter" should be thicker than pancake batter, but thinner than cooked oatmeal.

Tip on soaking nuts/seeds *Instead of soaking each nut and seed for its own specified amount of time, soak them together overnight. In this way they all get at least an 8 hour soak. Flax seeds, however, should be soaked on their own.*

Try your hand at creating your own cracker recipes!

Garlic Chili Flax Crackers

2 cups whole flax seeds

½ cup sesame seeds

3 cups water

4 garlic cloves

juice of 1 lemon

1 ½ tsp. sea salt

1 ½ tsp. onion powder

1 ½ tsp. chili powder

optional:

6 sun-dried tomato halves

1 fresh tomato

1 celery rib

PREP: Presoak flax and sesame seeds in water (3 cups, as indicated) for at least 4-6 hours. (Presoak sun-dried tomatoes for 1 hour, if using).

Process garlic cloves in food processor, then add lemon juice (amount to preference), sea salt, onion powder, chili powder and any optional ingredients. Mix into presoaked seeds. Spread thinly (about ¼ inch) on parchment paper. Dehydrate at 100 degrees for about 8-12 hours, until crisp. Flip crackers onto empty dehydrating tray and remove parchment paper midway through dehydration time. Store in refrigerator.

Garden Vegetable Flax Crackers

2 ½ cups whole flax seeds   1 ½ bell peppers

3 cups water   ¼ sweet/red onion

1 tomato   1 tsp. onion powder

2 celery ribs   1 tsp. sea salt

PREP: Presoak flax in water (3 cups, as indicated) for at least 4-6 hours.

Process chopped vegetables in food processor, then add sea salt and onion powder. Mix into presoaked seeds. Spread thinly (about ¼ inch) on parchment paper. Dehydrate at 100 degrees for about 8-12 hours, until crisp. Flip crackers onto empty dehydrating tray and remove parchment paper midway through dehydration time. Store in refrigerator.

Optional: Replace sweet onion with 4 green onions or a leek

Curried Flax Crackers

2 ½ cups whole flax seeds
3 cups water
4 garlic cloves
juice of ½ lemon
4 green onions
½ cup fresh parsley

1 ½ tsp. ground cumin
1 ½ tsp. onion powder
½ tsp. curry powder
1 Tbsp. turmeric
1 ½ tsp. sea salt
pinch cayenne (to taste)

PREP: Presoak flax in water (3 cups, as indicated) for at least 4-6 hours.

Process garlic cloves in food processor until minced. Add rest of ingredients (except for flax mixture) and up to 2 Tbsp. water to help with blending. Process until well-chopped. Mix into presoaked seeds. Spread thinly (about ¼ inch) on parchment paper. Dehydrate at 100 degrees for about 8-12 hours, until crisp. Flip crackers onto empty dehydrating tray and remove parchment paper midway through dehydration time. Store in refrigerator.

*The seasonings in this cracker are great
for combating candida!*

Tomato Herb Flax Crackers

2 cups whole flax seeds

½ cup sesame seeds

3 cups water

8 sun-dried tomato halves

1 tsp. chili powder

1 tsp. onion powder

½ tsp. garlic powder

1 tsp. paprika

$^{1}/_{8}$ - ¼ tsp. cayenne

2 tsp. dried oregano

2 tsp. dried basil

1 ½ tsp. sea salt

opt: ¼ cup dried onion

PREP: Presoak flax in water (3 cups, as indicated) for at least 4-6 hours.

Process sun-dried tomatoes and rest of ingredients (except for flax mixture and dried onions) in blender until smooth. Mix into presoaked seeds along with dried onion. Spread thinly (about ¼ inch) on parchment paper. Dehydrate at 100 degrees for about 8-12 hours, until crisp. Midway through dehydration time, flip crackers onto empty dehydrating tray and remove parchment paper. Store in refrigerator.

Optional: Add more herbs (oregano and basil) and cayenne for an even zippier flavor.

Onion Flax Crackers

2 ½ cups whole flax seeds

3 cups water

juice of 1 lemon

1 ½ tsp. sea salt

2 Tbsp. onion powder

1 ½ tsp. ground cumin

½ cup dried onion

PREP: Presoak flax in water (3 cups, as indicated) for at least 4-6 hours.

Mix lemon juice, sea salt, onion powder and cumin into soaked flax seeds. Mix dried onion in at the last possible moment before spreading onto parchment paper (or sprinkle spread mixture with dried onion). Dehydrate at 100 degrees for about 8-12 hours, until crisp. Flip crackers onto empty dehydrating tray and remove parchment paper midway through dehydration time. Store in refrigerator.

Garden Vegetable Cracker

1 ¼ cup whole flax seeds

3 cups sunflower seeds

¼ cup sesame seeds

6 sun-dried tomato halves

¼ sweet/red onion

1 carrot

1 celery rib

½ cup fresh parsley

1-2 garlic cloves

juice of ½ lemon

2 Tbsp. olive oil

1 tsp. dried basil

1 tsp. dried oregano

½ tsp. dried thyme

½ tsp. poultry seasoning

1 ½ tsp. sea salt

PREP: Presoak flax seed in 2 cups of water for at least 1-2 hours. Presoak sunflower seeds and sesame seeds at least 6 hours and sun-dried tomatoes for at least 1 hour.

Process vegetables in food processor until finely chopped. Add drained seeds and sun-dried tomatoes (not flax mixture), olive oil, lemon juice and a few tablespoons of water and process until well-mixed and finely chopped. In a bowl, mix ingredients from processor with flax mixture and herbs/seasonings. Spread about ¼ inch thick onto parchment paper on dehydrating trays. Cut into squares or diamonds by scoring lightly with a butter knife. Dehydrate for at least 12 hours, until crisp (flipping midway through dehydration time).

Sunflower Cracker

2 cups sunflower seeds	8 sun-dried tomato halves
¾ cup almonds	2 garlic cloves
¼ cup sesame seeds	2 tsp. apple cider vinegar
1 cup whole flax seeds	1 tsp. ground cumin
½ cup sweet/red onion	1 tsp. dried oregano
1 tomato	½ tsp. paprika
2 celery ribs	2 tsp. sea salt
½ red pepper	pinch cayenne

PREP: Presoak flax seed in 2 cups of water for at least 1-2 hours. Presoak sunflower seeds, almonds and sesame seeds for at least 8 hours. Presoak sun-dried tomatoes for 1 hour.

Drain soaked nut/seed mixture very well, then grind fairly fine in processor. Add to flax mixture. Add rest of ingredients to processor and puree well. Combine all together and then spread mixture about ¼ inch thick on parchment paper on dehydrator trays. Cut into squares or diamonds by scoring lightly with a butter knife. Dehydrate for at least 12 hours, until crisp. Flip crackers and remove parchment paper midway through dehydration time.

Veggie Crackers

1 cup dry whole peas (sprouted = about 1 quart)

4 carrots, shredded

¾ sweet/red onion

2 garlic cloves

½ cup tahini (pg. 100)

1 ½ tsp. sea salt

1 Tbsp. ground cumin

1 tsp. turmeric

juice of 1 lemon

PREP: Follow soaking/sprouting directions for whole peas.

Puree all ingredients together in food processor until smooth. Spread onto parchment paper (on dehydrator trays) about ¼ inch thick. Dehydrate at 100 degrees for at least 12-18 hours (until crisp and dry).   Flip crackers and remove parchment paper midway through dehydration time.

A similar recipe is made as a dip.
See directions on pg. 121.

Sunflower Cheese Crackers

Prepare **Sunflower Cheese** recipe on page 127. Spread about ¼ inch thick on parchment paper on dehydrating trays. Score with a knife into small squares. Dehydrate for at least 12 hours (until crisp). These are pretty close in flavor and texture to those familiar little orange cheese crackers many of us grew up with.

Nut Cheese Crackers

2 cups Brazil nuts   1 tsp. sea salt
juice of ½- 1 lemon

PREP: Presoak Brazil nuts for at least 8 hours

Process with juice of lemon and sea salt until smooth. Spread about ¼ inch thick on parchment paper on dehydrating trays. Score with a knife into small squares. Dehydrate for at least 12 hours (until crisp).

*Varying the amount of lemon juice determines
the sharpness of the "cheese".*

Pizza Crust

1 ½ cup buckwheat groats

1 cup sunflower seeds

½ - 1 tomato

6 sun-dried tomato halves

1 garlic clove

3 Tbsp. olive oil

1 tsp. honey

1 tsp. dried basil

1 tsp. dried oregano

1 tsp. sea salt

opt: 1 cup carrot pulp*

PREP: Soak 1 ½ cups buckwheat (equals 2 cups soaked) for at least 8 hours. Presoak sunflower seeds for at least 6 hours. Presoak sun-dried tomatoes for at least 1 hour.

Puree ingredients in left column in food processor. Add rest of ingredients (including carrot pulp) and process until well-mixed. Spread ¼-½ inch thick into 4-6 "personal-sized" pizza crusts onto parchment paper on dehydrating trays. Dehydrate about 24 hours, removing parchment paper midway through dehydration time.

* or grated carrots

Crummles* - a tasty crumbled topping

1 cup walnuts

1 cup sunflower seeds

½ cup pumpkin seeds

12 sun-dried tomato halves

¼ red/sweet onion

2 garlic cloves

½ red bell pepper

1 cup tomato soak water

1 Tbsp. olive oil

2 tsp. dried basil

2 tsp. dried oregano

2 tsp. ground cumin

½ tsp. poultry seasoning

1 tsp. sea salt

2 pinches of cayenne

PREP: Presoak walnuts for at least 4 hours, sunflower and pumpkin seeds for 6 hours, and sun-dried tomatoes for 1 hr.

Cut onion and pepper into small pieces so they process well. Process all ingredients in food processor until smooth. Roughly spread about ¼ inch thick onto a piece of parchment paper on a dehydrating tray. Dehydrate at 100 degrees for at least 10-12 hours, flipping and removing parchment paper midway through dehydration time. When fully dry, break into crumbles or chunks. *Great on salads, burritos and pizza!*

Some comment that it tastes like pepperoni. Not bad!

* *The creative name for this recipe is in honor of my father-in-law's unorthodox method of playing the game BOGGLE™.*

Curry Seasoned Seeds

3 cups seeds (pumpkin, or combo of pumpkin and sunflower)

1 ½ tsp. curry powder   1 - 2 tsp. turmeric

1 tsp. sea salt   1 ½ tsp. onion powder

¼ tsp. ground cumin   ½ tsp. garlic powder

PREP: Presoak seeds for at least 6-12 hours (overnight).

Drain seeds well and mix with seasonings. Spread on a sheet of parchment paper on a dehydrator tray. Dehydrate at 100 degrees for at least 18 hours. Flip from parchment paper onto another mesh tray midway through dehydration.

This tasty snack is a great choice
for those battling candida.

Chili Seasoned Seeds

3 cups seeds (pumpkin, or combo of pumpkin and sunflower)

½ red pepper	*1 tsp. ground cumin*
¼ tomato	*1 Tbsp. chili powder*
¼ sweet/red onion	*½ tsp. dried oregano*
4 sun-dried tomato halves	*$^1/_8$ tsp. cinnamon*
1 garlic clove	*¼ tsp. kelp powder*
$^1/_8$ tsp. cayenne	*¾ tsp. sea salt*

PREP: Presoak seeds for at least 6-12 hours (overnight). Separately presoak sun-dried tomatoes for at least 1 hour (drain before using).

Drain seeds well. Process rest of ingredients in food processor. Mix with seeds, then spread on a sheet of parchment paper on a dehydrator tray. Dehydrate at 100 degrees for at least 18 hours. Flip from parchment paper onto another mesh tray midway through dehydration. Break by hand into smaller pieces, if desired.

Pizza Seasoned Seeds

3 cups seeds (pumpkin, or combo of pumpkin and sunflower)

¼ tomato

$^1/_8$ sweet/red onion

4 sun-dried tomato halves

1 garlic clove

1 date, pitted

1 tsp. lemon juice

1 Tbsp. olive oil

½ tsp. onion powder

½ tsp. dried basil

1 ½ tsp. dried oregano

½ tsp. kelp powder

¾ tsp. sea salt

PREP: Presoak seeds for at least 6-12 hours (overnight). Presoak sun-dried tomatoes and date for at least 1 hour (drain before using).

Drain seeds well. Process rest of ingredients in food processor. Mix with seeds, then spread on a sheet of parchment paper on a dehydrator tray. Dehydrate at 100 degrees for at least 18 hours. Flip from parchment paper onto another mesh tray midway through dehydration. Break by hand into smaller pieces, if desired.

Mild Ranch Seasoned Seeds

3 cups seeds (pumpkin, or combo of pumpkin and sunflower)

¼ cup whole flax seeds   *1 tsp. dill weed*

*¾ cup **Garlic Ranch Dressing** (pg. 96)*   *¼ tsp. sea salt*

PREP: Presoak seeds for at least 6-12 hours (overnight).

Drain seeds well and mix with seasonings. Spread on a sheet of parchment paper on a dehydrator tray. Dehydrate at 100 degrees for at least 18 hours. Flip from parchment paper onto another mesh tray midway through dehydration.

Dehydrated Nuts

There are many benefits to soaking and dehydrating nuts. First of all, the soaking process improves the digestibility and nutritional profile of the nuts. Secondly, the texture and flavor of the nuts can be significantly changed. Thirdly, it's handy to have presoaked and dehydrated nuts ready for use in recipes that require "dry" nuts (like pie crusts). This process provides the dry nut texture but also offers the improved digestibility of soaked nuts.

I find pecans, in particular, are greatly improved by soaking and dehydrating. The bitter coating is removed and they are nice and crisp (more like a roasted nut).

Soak nuts for the amount of time specified in the **Soakables Chart** on pages 26-27. Drain and rinse, then spread in a single layer on a dehydrating sheet. Dehydrate for at least 24 hours to make sure they are completely dry.

Almonds, pecans and walnuts are some of our favorites to soak and dehydrate. Try these and others plain or coated with seasonings!

Salted Almonds

Presoak almonds. Rinse and drain well. Dissolve salt in a small amount of water and mix into almonds or sprinkle the almonds with finely ground sea salt. Spread on dehydrating tray and dehydrate until crisp (at least 18-24 hours).

Garlic Herb Almonds

2 cups almonds

10 garlic cloves

2 tsp. olive oil

2 Tbsp. water

1 Tbsp. honey

½ tsp. garlic powder

1 tsp. sea salt

1 tsp. dried basil

1 tsp. dried oregano

PREP: Presoak almonds at least 8 hours. Drain well.

Process garlic on its own in food processor. Add water, oil, honey, garlic powder and sea salt. Process until well mixed (can also blend in blender). Pour into a bowl. Mix in oregano, basil and drained almonds. Spread in a single layer on parchment paper on dehydrating sheets and dehydrate for at least 24-36 hours (until crisp).

Candied Pecans

2 cups pecans

3 Tbsp. honey

¼ tsp. cinnamon

¼ tsp. sea salt

PREP: Presoak pecans in water for at least 4 hours.

Rinse and drain pecans. Mix honey, 2 tsp. water, sea salt and cinnamon in a large bowl. Toss pecans in mixture, then spread on a piece of parchment paper on a dehydrating tray. Dehydrate at 100 degrees for about 24 hours, until crisp and not too gooey.

Candied Walnuts

2 cups walnuts

3 Tbsp. honey

¼ tsp. sea salt

opt: ¼ tsp. cinnamon

PREP: Presoak walnuts in water for at least 6 hours.

Rinse and drain walnuts. Mix honey, 2 tsp. water, and sea salt in a large bowl. Toss walnuts in mixture, then spread on a piece of parchment paper and follow the rest of the dehydration instructions above.

Orange Spice Almonds

2 cups almonds

¼ cup honey

¼ cup dates, pitted

zest of 1 orange

2 tsp. cinnamon

1 ½ tsp. pumpkin pie spice

¼ tsp. cloves

¼+ tsp. sea salt

PREP: Presoak almonds for at least 8 hours.

Process honey, dates, orange zest, spices and sea salt in blender or food processor until well-mixed. Mix with well-drained almonds. Spread in a single layer on parchment paper on dehydrating sheets and dehydrate for at least 24-36 hours (until crisp).

Simple Almond Cookies

1 ½ cup almonds

½ cup honey

pinch of sea salt

PREP: Presoak 1 ½ cup almonds for at least 8 hours

Grind almonds in food processor. Add sea salt and honey and process until smooth. Shape into cookies and place on dehydrating sheet. Dehydrate at least 8 hours.

Basic Cookie Recipe

Basic Cookie Dough

2 cups of a combination of sunflower seeds and nuts

¾ cup dates, pitted

½ - ¾ cup other dried fruit (raisins, apricots, figs, etc.)

1 - 3 tsp. spice (cinnamon, pumpkin pie spice, cardamom, etc.)

¼ tsp. sea salt

opt: fresh fruit (1-2 bananas, 1-2 apples, pineapple, mango)

Optional Mix-Ins (add after processing cookie dough)

½ - 1 cup chopped nuts (walnuts, pecans, almonds, etc.)

½ - 1 cup chopped dried fruit (raisins, dates, apricots, etc.)

PREP: Presoak seeds and nuts for at least 6-8 hours.

In food processor, process your choice of cookie dough ingredients until well-blended (add a small amount of water to mixture, if needed, for blendability). Mix in your choice of optional mix-ins. Drop by spoonful onto parchment paper on dehydrating trays and flatten to about ¼ inch thickness. Dehydrate at 100 degrees for 12-24 hours (until desired crispness).

Apple-Apricot Cookies

2 cups sunflower seeds/nuts

¾ cup dates, pitted

½ cup apricots

2 apples, peeled

2 tsp. lemon juice

2 tsp. cinnamon

¼ tsp. sea salt

½ cup chopped pecans

Process all ingredients, except for pecans, in food processor. Mix in pecans then follow directions on page 192.

Banana-Raisin Cookies

2 cups sunflower seeds/nuts

¾ cup dates, pitted

½ cup raisins

2 bananas

2 tsp. ground cardamom

1 tsp. cinnamon

¼ tsp. sea salt

½ cup chopped walnuts

Process all ingredients, except for walnuts, in food processor. Mix in walnuts then follow directions on page 192.

*My oldest son, John, helped create these cookie recipes using the **Basic Cookie Recipe**.*

Coconut Macaroons

1 coconut

½ cup dates, pitted

$^1/_3$ cup almonds

¼ cup honey

up to 1 cup water

pinch of sea salt

PREP: Presoak almonds for at least 8 hours (or use 2/3 cup presoaked almonds).

Remove meat from coconut and peel off dark outer skin. Process coconut in a food processor until shredded. Add rest of ingredients and blend until all is well-chopped and blended. Drop by mounds onto dehydrating trays. Watch the dehydration time on these- anywhere from 4-8 hours (it's nice to keep the center moist and outside crisp, like traditional macaroons).

These can also be prepared in a heavy-duty blender.
Just add all the ingredients and blend until well-mixed.

Banana Nut Cookies

2 cups Brazil nuts

3 bananas

¼ cup dates, pitted

½ tsp. ground cardamom

½ tsp. cinnamon

pinch of sea salt

PREP: Presoak Brazil nuts for at least 8 hours.

Process all ingredients (plus about ½ cup of water) in blender until smooth. Drop by spoonful onto parchment paper on dehydrating sheets (flatten until about ¼ inch thick) and dehydrate for at least 8 hours.

Cinnamon Nut Cookies

2 cups Brazil nuts

$^1/_3$ cup dates, pitted

1 tsp. cinnamon

pinch of sea salt

PREP: Presoak Brazil nuts for at least 8 hours.

Process all ingredients (and about 1 cup of water) in blender until smooth. Follow rest of instructions for recipe above.

Carob Cookies

¾ cup almonds

¾ cup sunflower seeds

¼ cup sesame seeds

²/₃ cup dates, pitted

¹/₃ cup raisins

3 Tbsp. honey

¼ tsp. sea salt

3 Tbsp. tahini (pg. 100)

½ cup carob powder

PREP: Presoak almonds for at least 8 hours. Sunflower seeds can be presoaked for at least 6 hours or ground along with sesame seeds with additional water added for ease in processing. Presoak raisins for at least 1 hour.

Grind sesame seeds then process soaked nuts and seeds and rest of ingredients until uniformly mixed. Shape into round flat cookies on parchment paper on dehydrating trays. Dehydrate for about 8 hours, flipping and removing parchment paper about halfway through time.

*These cookies can be made without a dehydrator-
just roll "dough" into balls and refrigerate
or freeze until ready to serve.*

Other Varieties of Carob Cookies

Carob Coconut Cookies

Add ½ cup coconut to cookie mixture in food processor.

Carob Mint Cookies – *our favorite version*

Add 1-2 tsp. peppermint extract or a few drops of peppermint oil to cookie mixture in food processor.

Carob Nut Cookies

Add ½ cup chopped nuts to already processed mixture before shaping into cookies on dehydrating trays.

Carob Raisin Cookies

Add ½ cup raisins to already processed mixture before shaping into cookies on dehydrating trays.

Plain cookies

Prepare cookie recipe and leave out tahini and carob powder.

Optional additions: *½ cup raisins   ½ cup chopped nuts*
½ tsp. pumpkin pie spice   ½ tsp. cinnamon

Shortbread Rice Cookies

1 cup sweet brown rice

$^1/_3$ cup water

¼ cup dates, pitted

1-2 Tbsp. honey

1 Tbsp. olive oil

16 presoaked almonds

¼ tsp. cinnamon

¼ tsp. pumpkin pie spice

$^1/_8$ tsp. sea salt

PREP: Soak and sprout 1 cup of sweet brown rice according to instructions in **Sproutables Chart** on page 27.

Process rice and rest of ingredients in heavy-duty blender. Spread about ¼ inch thick on parchment paper on dehydrating tray. Dehydrate until crisp (about 24 hours). Break into squares. The batter could also be dropped and spread into ¼ inch thick cookies before dehydrating.

Optional: Add ½ cup coconut to mixture before dehydrating.

Sweet Seed Cookies

1 cup sesame seeds

½ cup whole flax seeds

zest of 1 orange

juice of 2 oranges -

    plus water added

    to equal 1 ½ cups liquid

$^2/_3$ cup dates, pitted

$^1/_3$ cup raisins

2 Tbsp. honey

¼ tsp. cloves

¼ tsp. sea salt

PREP: Puree all but seeds together. Add to seeds in a large bowl and allow to sit for at least 4-6 hours.

Drop mixture onto parchment paper on dehydrating sheets by the spoonful, about ¼ inch thick. Dehydrate for at least 8-12 hours for a chewy cookie. Dehydrating longer can produce a nice, crisp cookie, especially when stored in refrigerator until ready to serve.

Optional additions: After soaking, mix in your choice of:

    3 mashed bananas

    2 grated apples

    ½ cup chopped nuts

Cereals

Grain-based cereals can be enjoyed any time of day-
as a meal or as a snack.

These cereal recipes feature buckwheat groats. This grain is versatile. It can simply be soaked prior to eating or soaked and dehydrated for a crisper cereal. (Raw oat groats can be substituted for the buckwheat, if desired. Rolled oats can be prepared into an excellent soaked cereal, yet rolled oats are usually steamed in processing, so are technically not raw).

This section includes recipes for:

> **Soaked cereals**
> **Porridges**
> **Dehydrated cereals**
> **Milks- for topping cereals**

Since there is so much flexibility in the creation of cereals,
be sure to record your favorite combinations!

Fruit and Nut Cereal

½ cup raw buckwheat groats
¼ - ½ cup dried fruit (raisins, dates, figs, apricots, etc.)
¼ - ½ cup nuts, seeds (almonds, pecans, walnuts, etc.)
Opt: 1-2 Tbsp. chia seeds (soaked with water on its own)

Cover the buckwheat, dried fruit and nuts/seeds with plenty of water and allow to soak for at least eight hours. Soak chia separately in ½-1 cup water for at least 1 hour. When ready to eat, rinse and drain buckwheat mixture thoroughly before adding a mashed banana, **Banana Milk** (pg. 202) and/or **Nut Milk** (pg. 203). Add presoaked chia, if including. The cereal can also be sprinkled with cinnamon, coconut, ground flax and fresh fruit or drizzled with a bit of honey, if desired.

An example of some great additions:

- 2 Tbsp. sunflower seeds
- ¼ cup almonds
- ¼ cup raisins
- 3 dates, chopped
- ½ banana, mashed
- a few fresh or frozen berries

Buckwheat Porridge

Prepare as for **Fruit and Nut Cereal** (pg. 201), but puree the soaked grains, fruits and nuts (after draining) with either orange juice or a banana (with some added water) in a blender before serving. Fresh fruit and berries are a nice addition. Additionally drizzle with honey and sprinkle with cinnamon before serving, if you'd like.

Excess buckwheat porridge can be spooned
onto dehydrating sheets and dehydrated
(for about 24 hours) into cookies.

Banana Milk

1 ½ bananas (frozen)   2 Tbsp. flax oil
2 cups water   opt: 1 date, pitted
pinch sea salt   or 1 tsp. honey

Puree in blender and use immediately over cereal or fruit salad.

This is a great milk alternative.
It's fast, easy and pleasantly sweet.

Almond Milk

½ cup almonds

3-4 dates, pitted

4 cups purified water

opt: pinch of sea salt

PREP: Soak almonds for at least 8 hours.

Drain and rinse almonds (remove skins from almonds if you want pure white milk) and then puree in blender with other ingredients. Strain, if desired. Keep refrigerated for up to 5 days.

Nut/Seed Milk

¼ cup almonds

Up to ¼ cup sunflower seeds

2 Tbsp. sesame seeds

3-4 dates, pitted

4 cups purified water

$^1/_8$ tsp. sea salt

PREP: Soak combination of nuts and seeds at least 8 hours.

Drain and rinse nuts/seeds (remove skins from almonds if you want pure white milk), then puree in blender with other ingredients. Strain, if desired. Refrigerate for up to 5 days.

Buckwheat Crunchies

Soak 2 cups of dry raw buckwheat groats in a quart jar or large bowl for at least 6-8 hours. Rinse and drain well (gelatinous liquid forms on soaking buckwheat). Spread on parchment paper (on dehydrator tray) and then dehydrate at 100 degrees for 6-8 hours (until crisp).

Add dehydrated cereal to a bowl with any desired dried fruit or fresh fruit and/or nuts and then top with **Banana Milk** (pg. 202) or **Nut Milk** (pg. 203).

This is the simplest way to prepare and enjoy this cereal.
You can also add an assortment of other ingredients
before dehydrating to provide some variety.
You can arrive at new tasty combinations on your own
or try some of the recipes on the following page.

Buckwheat is a really neat, unique grain. In fact, it is technically not a grain but the seed of an herb. Many assume that it is related to wheat because of its name, yet buckwheat is no relation to wheat and contains no gluten.

Other Varieties of Buckwheat Crunchies

Cinnamon Crunchies

$^{1}/_{3}$ cup honey   2 pinches of sea salt

½ tsp. cinnamon   (opt: pinch pumpkin pie spice)

Mix drained quart of presoaked buckwheat (pg. 204) with ingredients above. Dehydrate for at least 6-8 hours.

Optional: Presoak ¼ cup sesame seeds and mix with buckwheat and honey mixture before dehydrating.

Carob/Cocoa Crunchies

Follow recipe for **Cinnamon Crunchies** (above), except additionally add 3-4 Tbsp. of carob powder or 2 Tbsp. cacao powder to mixture.

Apple Cinnamon Crunchies

Blend 1 apple, 1-2 tsp. lemon juice and an additional 1 tsp. of cinnamon with the ingredients for **Cinnamon Crunchies** (above).

Granola

4 cups buckwheat groats	$^2/_3$ cup sunflower seeds
½ cup almonds	1 cup nuts
½ cup honey	
$^1/_3$ cup dates, pitted	
3 Tbsp. coconut or olive oil	**after dehydration:**
¼ cup water	1 cup raisins
1 Tbsp. cinnamon	¾ cup dates, figs,
1 tsp. sea salt	apricots, etc.

PREP: Presoak buckwheat groats and ½ cup of almonds for 8- 12 hours. Separately presoak sunflower seeds and 1 cup of nuts- your choice of walnuts, pecans, almonds, etc.

Rinse and drain buckwheat and add to a large bowl. In blender, process rest of ingredients in left column until smooth, then add to bowl. Chop the 1 cup of soaked nuts and add along with sunflower seeds to bowl with buckwheat. Mix well. Spread on parchment paper on dehydrating trays and dehydrate at 100 degrees for at least 24 hours (you want these good and crisp so they are easy to chew). Mix in dried fruit when done.

*Serve with **Banana Milk** (pg. 202) for a traditional treat!*

Other Varieties of Granola

Banana Nut Granola

Blend 2-3 bananas into sauce mixture and add more chopped nuts before dehydrating.

Apple Cinnamon Granola

Blend 2 apples and more cinnamon (to taste) with sauce mixture before mixing with grains.

Tropical Granola

Add ½ cup shredded coconut to grains before dehydrating plus chopped dried pineapple, mango and/or papaya (unsulphured, unsweetened) after dehydrating.

Desserts and Treats

Desserts and Treats, cont.

Desserts and Treats, cont.

Desserts can be enjoyed **following a meal,** on their own **as a snack** or even as an occasional **full meal**!
For a **dessert dinner**, try any combination of:

Fruit smoothie	Ice cream	Raw pies
Fruit salad	Stuffed dates	Truffles

Be sure to reference the **Fruit Section** for other great dessert and treat recipes like Stuffed Dates, Fruit Smoothies and Fruit Salad, and the **Snack/Dehydrates** section for cookies, candied nuts, etc.

In terms of food-combining principles, it's always best to wait 1-2 hours after a meal before eating a fruit-based dessert.

Soft-Serve Ice Cream

8-10 frozen bananas   ¾ cup almonds
2-3 cups frozen fruit   or walnuts

Using the blank attachment (not screen) in a masticating juicer, alternatively process bananas, fruit and nuts into a bowl. Stir well and enjoy! Delicious topped with chopped fresh fruit and/or nuts.

Strawberry Ice Cream- use frozen strawberries

Blueberry Ice Cream- use frozen blueberries

Peach Ice Cream- use frozen peaches

Mango Ice Cream- use frozen mangos

Banana Ice Cream- omit frozen fruit, use more bananas

Cinnamon Raisin Ice Cream- add ½-1 cup of soaked
    raisins in place of frozen fruit and up to 2 tsp. cinnamon.

Cookie Dough Ice Cream- make Banana Ice Cream and
    mix in small pieces of **Date Nut Pie Crust** (pg. 227).

*People are always amazed at how this dairy and sugar-free
ice cream is so deliciously rich and creamy!*

Ice Cream Pie

Pour **Soft-serve Ice Cream** (pg. 211) into a **Date Nut Pie Crust** (pg. 227) and place in freezer just until firm enough to serve (1-2 hours).

Optional: Reserve some crust and crumble on top of filling before freezing.

Variation: Prepare this same pie with **Fruit Smoothie** (pg. 58) as the filling in place of the Soft-serve Ice Cream.

Banana Split

Soft-serve Ice Cream *(pg. 211)*

Bananas

plus any combination of the following toppings:

carob sauce	*glazed bananas*
chopped strawberries	*chopped pineapple*
chopped nuts	*chopped mango*
shredded coconut	*ground flax*

Slice a banana lengthwise.   Place in bowl.   Top with **Soft-serve Ice Cream** (pg. 211).   Drizzle with **Carob Sauce** (pg. 217) and sprinkle with chopped strawberries, pineapple, nuts, etc.

Carob Shake

$^{1}/_{3}$ cup almonds

1 ¼ cup water

3-4 dates, pitted

2 Tbsp. tahini (pg. 100)

1 Tbsp. flax oil

3 Tbsp. carob powder*

3 frozen bananas

pinch sea salt

Process almonds, dates and water in blender until smooth. Add rest of ingredients and blend only until smooth (still want it to be frosty like a shake). *If you have presoaked almonds on hand, you can replace the 1/3 cup dry almonds with about ½ cup presoaked almonds. * or 2 Tbsp. cacao powder*

Variation: Carob Pops Pour into pop molds and freeze.

Almond Butter Fudge

2 cups almonds

½ cup dates, pitted

¼ cup raisins

1 Tbsp. flax oil

2 Tbsp. honey

¼ tsp. sea salt

Process all ingredients in food processor until quite smooth (this will take a while). Press into small pan, then cut into squares. Refrigerate until ready to serve.

Carob Tahini Candy

$^1/_3$ cup tahini (pg. 100)   ¼ cup carob powder

¼ cup honey   pinch sea salt

Hand mix ingredients together in a bowl. Roll into small balls and put in freezer until ready to serve.

Variation: Before rolling into balls, add your choice of shredded coconut, chopped nuts, raisins, sesame seeds, etc. **Optional:** For carob-mint flavor add peppermint extract.

This recipe is handy because it's so quick to prepare.

Raisin Nut Clusters

$^1/_3$ - ½ cup carob powder $^1/_3$ cup coconut oil

2 Tbsp. honey   2 pinches sea salt

2 Tbsp. tahini (pg. 100)   ¾ cup raisins

½ cup dates, pitted   ½ cup walnuts/pecans

Mix all ingredients, except raisins and nuts, in food processor until smooth. This will be a bit messy and works best if coconut oil is slightly softened.   Hand-mix in raisins and nuts. Drop and freeze into candy clusters.

Valentine Candies

½ cup coconut oil
¾ cup dates, pitted
¼ cup honey

3 Tbsp. carob powder
pinch of sea salt
¾ cup chopped nuts

Mix all but nuts in food processor. Be careful to not over-process. (Add 1 Tbsp. water if the mixture separates). This will be a bit messy- works best if coconut oil is slightly softened. Mix in nuts, then spread in an 8 x 8 pan. Refrigerate and cut into small squares.

*This candy was developed on Valentine's day
for my sweethearts!*

Honey Sesame Treats

1 ½ cup sesame seeds
¼ cup walnuts or pecans
1-2 pinches of sea salt

1 Tbsp. tahini (pg. 100)
$^1/_3$ cup honey
opt: $^1/_3$ cup coconut

In food processor, process sesame seeds and nuts into a coarse meal (some seeds still whole). Add sea salt, tahini and honey, and process until mixture begins to hold together. Press into a small pan, refrigerate, then cut into squares.

Variation: Add 3 Tbsp. carob powder.

Peppermint Candy

1 coconut	3-4 Tbsp. carob powder
4 Tbsp. honey	pinch of sea salt
½-1 tsp. peppermint extract	

Simple Version Remove meat from coconut. Peel off dark outer skin. Finely chop coconut in food processor. Add rest of ingredients and process until well-mixed. Press into a small pan. Refrigerate and then cut into small squares.

Layered Version Prepare chopped coconut as described above. Remove half of the coconut from processor to a bowl. To coconut in processor add peppermint extract and ½ of honey (2 Tbsp.). Mix and place in another bowl. Place other half of coconut into processor and add rest of honey (2 Tbsp.), carob powder and pinch of sea salt. Press half of this mixture into bottom of small pan. Press white coconut mixture on top of this and finish by pressing rest of carob coconut mixture on top. This makes a beautiful layered presentation.

A smoother, hold-together consistency can be achieved by blending the ingredients in a heavy-duty blender instead of using a food processor. Be careful to not overblend/overheat.

Carob Sauce

1 cup pitted dates*   3 Tbsp. tahini (pg. 100)
¼ cup raisins   3 Tbsp. nut butter
¼ cup coconut oil $^1/_8$ tsp. sea salt
$^1/_3$ cup carob powder $^2/_3$ cup water

PREP: Presoak dates and raisins for at least 20 minutes. Drain and then process until smooth with the rest of the ingredients in a heavy duty blender.

* or substitute ¼ cup (or more) of honey for ½ cup of the dates, reducing the amount of water slightly.

Great for drizzling over smoothies, shakes
and **Soft-serve Ice Cream** (pg. 211).

You can also dip frozen bananas in this sauce before sprinkling them with chopped nuts or shredded coconut.

Fudge

$^1/_3$ cup pumpkin seeds

$^1/_3$ cup walnuts/pecans

2 Tbsp. tahini (pg. 100)

2-3 Tbsp. honey

$^1/_3$ cup carob powder

2 Tbsp. raisins

$^1/_3$ cup dates, pitted

pinch of sea salt

_____

½ cup chopped nuts

Briefly rinse raisins with boiling water. Finely grind pumpkin seeds and the 1/3 cup walnuts or pecans in food processor. Add rest of ingredients (except for chopped nuts) and process until very smooth (forming an oily-looking ball in the processor). Mix in chopped nuts and press into small pan. Refrigerate, then cut into squares when ready to serve.

Optional: Use sunflower seeds in place of pumpkin seeds.
Variation: Add 1/3 cup coconut with or in place of chopped nuts.

Lemon Squares

Crust ingredients

¾ cup almonds

½ cup pecans

½ cup walnuts

½ cup dates, pitted

3 Tbsp. honey

¾ cup shredded coconut

1-2 pinches of sea salt

Topping ingredients

1 cup dates, pitted

¾ cup walnuts

¼ cup honey

zest from 1 lemon

juice of 1 lemon*

pinch of sea salt

1+ tsp. psyllium powder

PREP: Presoak dates and walnuts listed under topping ingredients for at least 2 hours.

Crust: Process almonds into a meal in food processor. Process with rest of crust ingredients in processor until the mixture begins to hold together.   Press into a small rectangular baking pan.

Topping: Drain soaked dates and walnuts and then process with rest of the topping ingredients in a food processor until smooth. Let mixture sit for a few minutes and then process again (to work out any psyllium lumps). Spread onto crust. Sprinkle top with additional coconut, if desired.

for a tangier bar add the juice of an additional lemon plus an additional teaspoon of psyllium powder.

Basic Cake Recipe

1 cup walnuts

1 cup pecans

$^2/_3$ cup almonds

2 apples

juice of 1 orange

1 cup dates, pitted

2 Tbsp. honey

2 tsp. cinnamon

pinch of sea salt

1 cup chopped dried fruit

    (raisins, figs, apricots, etc.)

opt: additional chopped nuts

In food processor, finely chop nuts (some should be ground and some in larger pieces). Remove to a large bowl. Add peeled and cored apples, orange juice, dates, honey, cinnamon and sea salt to food processor and process until smooth. Add this mixture and chopped dried fruit to ground nuts. Mix well, then shape into a round or square cake on a serving plate. Refrigerate for at least 2-3 hours before serving. Top with frosting or simply slice and serve.

Banana Version

Replace apples with bananas and up to 1/3 cup water for orange juice. Add 1 tsp. cardamom and another teaspoon of cinnamon.

Other Versions of Cake Recipe

Holiday Fruit Cake

Add zest from 1 lemon and 1 orange. Add at least (to taste) 1 tsp. ground cardamom, ¼ tsp. ground cloves plus another teaspoon of cinnamon. Add more chopped nuts and additional chopped dried fruits- any combination of figs, dates, raisins, apricots, pineapple, etc.. Press into a loaf pan. Refrigerate for at least 8-12 hours before slicing and serving.

Carrot Cake

Finely grate 1-2 carrots and add to cake mixture.

Add ½-1 cup of coconut, if desired.

Optional: Replace apples with pineapple.

Tropical Cake

Substitute pineapple and/or mango for apples.

Add ½-1 cup of coconut, if desired.

Carob Cake

Add 1/3-½ cup carob powder and 2 Tbsp. tahini

Frosting

1 ¼ cup dates, pitted   2 Tbsp. coconut or olive oil

¾ cup walnuts   pinch sea salt

2-4 Tbsp. honey

PREP: Presoak dates and walnuts for at least 6 hours.

Process all ingredients (and any optional additions from below) in food processor until smooth and fluffy. (Add a tablespoon of water at a time for a thinner consistency).

Optional additions:

   1-2 Tbsp. lemon juice (for a cream cheese-style frosting)

   zest from one orange or lemon

   2 Tbsp. carob powder

Frozen Layer Cake

½ cup almonds

6 - 7 bananas

¼ cup dates, pitted

2 cups figs, destemmed

2 cups dates, pitted

1 ½ cup chopped nuts

PREP: Presoak almonds for at least 8 hours.

Choose a shallow bowl or cake pan in which to build the layer cake. Rinse the dried fruit in the right column with boiling water, then soak in water for a few minutes. Drain dried fruit then add to a food processor and pulse process until just chopped. Process ingredients in left column in blender until smooth. Sprinkle bottom of bowl/pan with ½ cup of the chopped nuts (your choice of walnuts, pecans, almonds, etc.). Press about 1/3 of fig/date mixture on top of nuts. Pour about 1/3 of blended mixture over dried fruit layer. Sprinkle with nuts, press on dried fruit mixture, and pour on banana mixture- then repeat once more. Cover and freeze this layer cake for at least 8 hours before slicing and serving.

This layer cake is a nice option for holidays, birthdays and other special occasions.

Frozen Pies

All these frozen banana-based pies can be made in a heavy-duty blender (as indicated in recipes) or prepared in a juicer.

For making with a juicer: Begin with all frozen ingredients and alternate ingredients as you push them through the juicer. Mix briefly and pour into pie crust before freezing.

Freeze pies for at least 1-2 hours.

Before serving: Take out of freezer and leave at room temperature for 10-15 minutes or place in refrigerator for about ½ hour. This will allow the pie to soften slightly so it is easier to slice.

Banana Cream Pie

2 fresh bananas $^2/_3$ cup dates, pitted
4 frozen bananas

Process fresh bananas and dates in a heavy-duty blender. Add frozen bananas and process just until well-mixed (want to keep as frozen as possible). Pour into crust (**Date Nut Crust** (pg. 277) and **Carob Crust** (pg. 228) work well with this pie) and place in freezer for at least 1-2 hours before serving.

Coconut Banana Cream Pie

2 fresh bananas

4 frozen bananas

$^2/_3$ cup dates, pitted

1 cup shredded coconut

Process fresh bananas and dates in a heavy-duty blender. Add frozen bananas and process just until well-mixed (want to keep as frozen as possible). Add coconut (reserve a small amount) and pour into crust (**Date Nut Crust** (pg. 277) and **Carob Crust** (pg. 228) work well with this pie). Sprinkle top with coconut before freezing.

Carob Mint Pie

2 fresh bananas

4 frozen bananas

$^1/_3$ cup dates, pitted

½ cup presoaked almonds

¼ cup carob powder

½ - 1 tsp. peppermint extract

opt: 2 Tbsp. tahini (pg. 100)

Process fresh bananas and rest of ingredients (except frozen bananas) in a heavy-duty blender. Add frozen bananas and process just until well-mixed (want to keep as frozen as possible). Pour into crust (**Carob Pie Crust** (pg. 228) is great with this pie) and place in freezer for at least 1-2 hours before serving.

Pie Crust Options

Almond Date Pie Crust-

  Simple, easy to make, versatile

Date Nut Pie Crust-

  Sweet and rich, great for holiday pies

Carob Pie Crust-

  Perfect for frozen pies

Smooth Pie Crust-

  Prepared with presoaked almonds

Simple Pie Crust-

  Easy and tasty (included in Truffle section of book, pg. 236)

Press any of these into the base and sides of a pie pan.

Almond Date Pie Crust

1 ½ cup almonds (can substitute ½ cup pecans or walnuts)
¾ cup dates, pitted   pinch sea salt

Process in food processor until finely chopped and holds together when pinched. A small amount of honey can be added if it isn't holding together well enough.

Date Nut Pie Crust (and Cookies)

1 cup pecans

1 cup walnuts

1 cup dates, pitted

¼ - ½ cup honey (to taste)

¼ - ½ tsp. sea salt (to taste)

Grind pecans, walnuts and dates in food processor until well-chopped and blended. Add honey and continue to process until mixture forms a ball. *Be careful to not over-process.*

For a pie crust:

Press into base and sides of pie pan before adding filling. Reserve some of the mixture to crumble on top of the finished pie.

As cookies/truffles:

Optional additions:

> 1 tsp. cinnamon or pumpkin pie spice
>
> or 1 Tbsp. carob powder or cacao powder
>
> or 1-2 Tbsp. orange zest

Roll the dough into balls, then roll in flaked coconut, ground nuts, carob/cacao powder or sesame seeds.

These cookies make excellent holiday treats and presents.

Carob Pie Crust

½ cup sunflower seeds

½ cup almonds

½ cup walnuts or pecans

1 Tbsp. tahini (pg. 100)

2-4 Tbsp. carob powder

½ cup dates, pitted

¼ cup raisins

2 Tbsp. honey

pinch of sea salt

Briefly rinse raisins with boiling water. Process seeds and nuts in food processor until finely chopped. Add rest of ingredients and process until well-mixed, but not over-processed. Should hold together when pinched between your fingers. Press into a pie pan (or form into cookie balls).

Especially good with banana-based frozen pies.

Smooth Pie Crust

¾ cup almonds

½ cup walnuts/pecans

¼+ cup dates, pitted

$^1/_3$ cup raisins

PREP: Presoak almonds for at least 8 hours.

Grind all ingredients in food processor until ball forms. Press into bottom and sides of pie plate.

Optional-Line crust with sliced bananas before adding filling.

Strawberry Pie

2 pints of strawberries

$^2/_3$ cup dates, pitted

4 tsp. psyllium powder

Process one half pint of strawberries with dates and psyllium powder until quite smooth. Chop rest of strawberries and combine with strawberry/date mixture. Pour into prepared crust. Refrigerate until firm (at least ½ hour).

   Almond Date Crust (pg. 226) is quite good with this pie.

Strawberry Apple Pie

1 pint strawberries (½ to puree, ½ to chop)

1 apple

¼ cup dates, pitted

2 tsp. lemon juice

2 tsp. psyllium

Puree half of berries plus apple, dates, and lemon juice in processor. Add psyllium, process and then let sit for a few minutes. Chop rest of berries into a bowl. Puree mixture again. Mix with chopped berries then add filling to crust. Refrigerate until firm (at least ½ hour).

   Almond Date Crust (pg. 226) and
Smooth Pie Crust (pg. 228) are good options with this pie.

Apple Pie

4 Granny Smith apples	¼ tsp. sea salt
2 sweet apples	1 tsp. psyllium powder
¼ cup honey	4 dates, pitted
2 tsp. cinnamon	1 cup raisins

PREP: Prepare 1 batch of **Date Nut Pie Crust** (pg. 227) and press into pie plate as crust. Reserve a small amount to sprinkle on top of finished pie.

Peel apples. In food processor, puree 3 Granny Smith apples and 1 sweet apple with honey, cinnamon, sea salt, dates and psyllium powder into an applesauce consistency. Allow to sit for a couple of minutes, then reprocess (to work out any psyllium lumps). Pour mixture into a bowl. Mix in raisins. In processor, coarse chop last two apples. Mix into bowl. Ideally allow the pie filling to sit for about ½ hour before adding to crust so the raisins have a chance to absorb some of the excess moisture. Pour into crust, smooth top and sprinkle with reserved crust topping. Refrigerate until ready to serve.

Optional: Add ½ cup chopped walnuts to pie filling.

Mince Pie

5 apples	½ - 1 tsp. ground cloves
$^1/_3$ cup dates, pitted	¼ tsp. nutmeg
grated rind of 1 orange	¼ tsp. sea salt
juice of 1 orange	1 tsp. psyllium powder
$^1/_3$ cup honey	1 ½ cup raisins
1 Tbsp. cinnamon	½ cup chopped walnuts

PREP: Prepare 1 batch of **Date Nut Pie Crust** (pg. 227) and press into pie plate as crust for the pie. Reserve a small amount to sprinkle on top of finished pie.

Peel all five apples. Put 3 of the apples plus the rest of the ingredients (except for the raisins, walnuts and 2 reserved apples) in a food processor and process until smooth. Wait for a couple of minutes and process once more (in case there are any lumps) then pour into a bowl. Use food processor to chop 2 remaining apples and raisins, then add to bowl. Add walnuts to bowl. Allow all ingredients to sit in bowl for several hours- for spices to deepen and raisins and nuts to absorb extra liquid. Before serving, pour filling into pie crust.

A lovely pie for the holidays!

Sweet Potato Pie

½ cup macadamia nuts

1/3-½ cup honey, to taste

¼ tsp. sea salt

1 ½ tsp. cinnamon

½ tsp. pumpkin pie spice

juice of 1 orange

rind of $^1/_8$ of orange

5 sweet potatoes, peeled

2 tsp. psyllium powder

$^1/_3$ cup raisins

PREP: Presoak macadamias for 2-4 hours. Prepare **Date Nut Pie Crust** (pg. 227) and press into pie plate for crust. Reserve some to sprinkle on finished pie.

Drain macadamias, then puree all but sweet potatoes, psyllium and raisins in a heavy-duty blender. Cut sweet potatoes into chunks and add to blender, processing until smooth. Add psyllium, blend well and allow to sit for a few minutes. Blend again (until smooth). Sprinkle raisins on crust, then pour in filling. Sprinkle reserved **Date Nut** mixture on top. Refrigerate until ready to serve.

Pudding version- Serve in bowls (with no crust).

Casserole version- Add soaked dried fruit, fresh chunked pineapple, etc. and serve in a casserole dish.

Pumpkin Pie

1 pie pumpkin (about 4-5 cups, peeled and chunked)

½ cup walnuts, Brazil nuts, macadamias or coconut

¾ cup almonds   ½ tsp. ground ginger

1 avocado   ¼ tsp. ground nutmeg

$^1/_3$ cup honey   ½ tsp. sea salt

¼ cup dates, pitted   1 tsp. psyllium powder

1 tsp. cinnamon   1 cup raisins

PREP: Presoak nuts for at least 8 hours. Prepare **Date Nut Pie Crust** (pg. 227) and press into pie plate for crust.

Process drained nuts, avocado, honey, dates, spices, sea salt and psyllium until smooth. Slowly add chunks of pumpkin and keep processing until very smooth. Mix in raisins and pour into crust, smoothing top with a spatula. Refrigerate until ready to serve.

Cranapple Cheesecake

Cranapple Layer

1 cup cranberries

¼ dates, pitted

1 apple, cored

$^1/_3$ cup honey

¼ tsp. sea salt

1 Tbsp. orange zest

Cheesecake Topping

2 cups macadamias*

$^1/_3$ cup honey

juice of 1 lemon

¼ tsp. sea salt

PREP: Presoak macadamias for 2-4 hours. Prepare **Date Nut Pie Crust** (pg. 227) and press into pie plate for crust.

Process cranapple layer ingredients in food processor until well chopped and blended. Spread onto pie crust. Puree cheesecake topping ingredients in heavy-duty blender until smooth. Spread onto pie. Refrigerate until ready to serve.

For a more economical option (though not technically as raw), substitute 2 cups of presoaked raw cashews and 1/3 cup coconut oil for the macadamias.

Variation: Reverse order of layers, if desired.

Rich! This reminds me of the not-so-good-for-you no-bake cherry cheesecake my mom has made for years.

Strawberry Cheesecake

Strawberry Topping

1 pint strawberries

¼ cup dates, pitted

opt: fresh blueberries

Cheesecake Filling

2 cups macadamias*

$^1/_3$ cup honey

juice of 1 lemon

¼ tsp. sea salt

PREP: Presoak macadamias for 2-4 hours. Prepare **Date Nut Pie Crust** (pg. 227) and press into pie plate for crust.

Puree cheesecake topping ingredients in heavy-duty blender until smooth. Pour into pie crust. Process half of strawberries with dates. Chop rest of strawberries and mix with strawberry/date sauce. Pour over top of pie filling. Sprinkle with blueberries. Refrigerate until ready to serve.

For a more economical option (though technically not as raw), substitute 2 cups of presoaked raw cashews and 1/3 cup coconut oil for the macadamias.

This makes a great birthday treat!

Fruit and Nut-based Truffles

These tasty treats made simply from a combination of dried fruit and nuts **are a great raw food staple**.   Truffles like these are a great substitute for traditional cookies and candies.   Enjoy trying the recipes here as well as creating your own combinations.

Truffle and **Pie Crust** recipes are pretty much interchangeable since they're both prepared from dried fruit and nuts with the optional addition of honey and spices. Any great-tasting truffle recipe can be pressed into a pie plate as a pie crust. *Give it a try!*

Simple Truffles (and Pie Crust)

Equal parts: *almonds*   *walnuts*   *dates*

Process ingredients in food processor until the mixture begins forming a ball. Press into a pie plate or roll into balls.
Optional: Add a pinch of sea salt before combining.

Basic Truffles

1 cup raisins $^2/_3$ cup dates, pitted
$^2/_3$ cup almonds $^1/_3$ cup walnuts

Briefly rinse raisins with boiling water (or add up to 2 Tbsp. of water to mixture in food processor). Chop almonds briefly before adding the rest of the ingredients and then process until coarsely ground and starting to hold together (forming a ball in processor). Roll into small balls, then roll in sesame seeds, carob powder, chopped nuts or coconut. Refrigerate until ready to serve.

Spiced Truffles

1 cup almonds   ¾- 1 tsp. pumpkin pie spice
¼ cup sesame seeds $^1/_8$ tsp. sea salt
1 cup dates, pitted

Process almonds and sesame seeds in food processor until finely chopped. Continue processing after adding dates, spice and sea salt until mixture starts to hold together. Form into balls and refrigerate before serving.
Optional: Roll balls in sesame seeds.

Apricot Nut Truffles

½ cup raisins

½ cup dates, pitted

½ cup apricots

½ cup almonds

½ cup walnuts

or pecans

Briefly rinse raisins and apricots with boiling water. Chop nuts and almonds briefly in food processor before adding dried fruit, then process until coarsely ground and starting to hold together (forming a ball in processor). Roll into small balls, then roll in sesame seeds, carob powder, chopped nuts or coconut. Refrigerate until ready to serve.

Date Coconut Truffles

1 cup dates, pitted

1 cup raisins

$^2/_3$ cup nuts (your choice)

1- 1 ½ cups coconut

Briefly rinse dried fruit with boiling water. Grind nuts in food processor, then continue to process with dried fruit and ¾ cup of coconut until mixture holds together. Roll into balls, then roll to coat in remaining coconut.

Fig Nut Truffles

1 cup figs

½ cup raisins

½ cup dried apricots

$^2/_3$ cup walnuts/pecans

opt: $^2/_3$ cup coconut

Briefly rinse raisins and apricots with boiling water. Destem figs, tear in half and check for quality. Place with raisins, apricots, nuts (and coconut- reserving some for rolling) in food processor and process until everything is uniformly chopped (but not pureed). Roll into balls and refrigerate. **Optional:** Roll balls in coconut.

Fruit and Nut Truffles

1 cup almonds

¾ cup pecans or walnuts

¾ cup raisins

¾ cup dates, pitted

¼ cup orange juice

½ cup coconut

Pulse nuts and dried fruits in processor into a coarse meal. Add juice and pulse until mixture begins forming into a ball. Roll into balls and then roll in coconut.

Melt-In-Your-Mouth Truffles

¾ cup almonds   ½ cup raisins

½ cup walnuts   ½ tsp. cinnamon

1/3- ½ cup dates, pitted   pinch sea salt

PREP: Presoak almonds and walnuts (at least 6-8 hours).

Process all ingredients together in food processor until well-chopped (but not smooth).   Roll into balls, then roll in coconut, sesame seeds, chopped nuts or carob powder.

*What distinguishes these truffles from others is that the nuts
are presoaked. This is preferential in terms of digestibility,
yet changes the texture and flavor of the final product.
They are moister and have a milder flavor.*

Index

*Recipes in **bold type** are*

good basic recipes and proven family favorites

A

B

D

P

Q, R

S

T

U, V

W

X, Y, Z